RESPIRATION

D1441093

Paul Berghuis, DO
Chief Resident, Anesthesiology
Clinical Instructor, Anesthesiology
Dartmouth-Hitchcock Medical Center
Hanover, New Hampshire 03756

Neal Cohen, MD, MPH, MS
Department of Anesthesiology and Critical Care
University of San Francisco Hospital
San Francisco, California 94143

Michael Decker, CRTT
Senior Research Assistant
Pulmonary and Critical Care Medicine
University Hospitals of Cleveland
Cleveland, Ohio 44106

Andrew Gettinger, MD
Assistant Professor of Anesthesiology
Medical Director, Critical Care Service
Dartmouth-Hitchcock Medical Center
Hanover, New Hampshire 03756

Kenneth Myrabo, RRT, MED
Manager of Respiratory Care Services
University of Washington Medical Center
Seattle, Washington 98195

Jon Nilsestuen, PhD, RRT
Associate Professor & Program Director
Department of Respiratory Care
University of Texas Health Science Center
Houston, Texas 77225

Kingman Strohl, MD
Chief, Pulmonary and Critical Care Medicine
University Hospitals of Cleveland
Cleveland, Ohio 44106

John Yount, MD
Oregon Health Sciences
Portland, Oregon 97201

© SpaceLabs, Inc., 1992

All rights reserved

No part of this book may be reproduced by any means,
or transmitted, or translated into a machine language
without the written permission of the publisher.

All brands and product names are trade marks of their
respective owners.

Published by SpaceLabs, Inc., Redmond, Washington, U.S.A.

Printed in the United States

ISBN 0-9627449-3-X

TABLE OF CONTENTS

TABLE OF CONTENTS

TABLE OF CONTENTS

INTRODUCTION

To provide the best possible diagnosis, today's clinicians need to understand both the capabilities and limitations of medical devices which measure respiration. In this book, Section 1.0 reviews the physiologic function of the respiratory system. The section includes a discussion of the physical laws that apply to gases and gas exchange. Section 2.0 outlines the mechanical principles that govern the volume, flow, and pressure of gases in monitoring devices used in the clinical environment.

Section 3.0 describes the principles used in pulse oximetry technology, which has grown in use to assess patient arterial oxygenation and gas exchange. Section 4.0 discusses the techniques for measuring the oxygen saturation of mixed venous oxygen. By monitoring the mixed venous oxygen saturation, clinicians can better manage cardiorespiratory problems.

Section 5.0 presents the current state of impedance pneumography in the detection of respiratory effort, particularly in neonatal and pediatric intensive care units. This section also discusses improvements to impedance pneumography now under investigation. Section 6.0 outlines the measurement principles of anesthesia gases and carbon dioxide. Capnography has proven beneficial in monitoring patients during general anesthesia.

The monitoring of respiration requires the measurement of various parameters from several physiologic viewpoints. This book attempts to place each method and its associated devices in perspective so that patient care can be enhanced.

Figure 1.1— The respiratory system consists of an upper airway (including the nasal cavity, oral cavity, pharynx, and larynx) and a lower airway (consisting of a trachea, right, and left lungs).

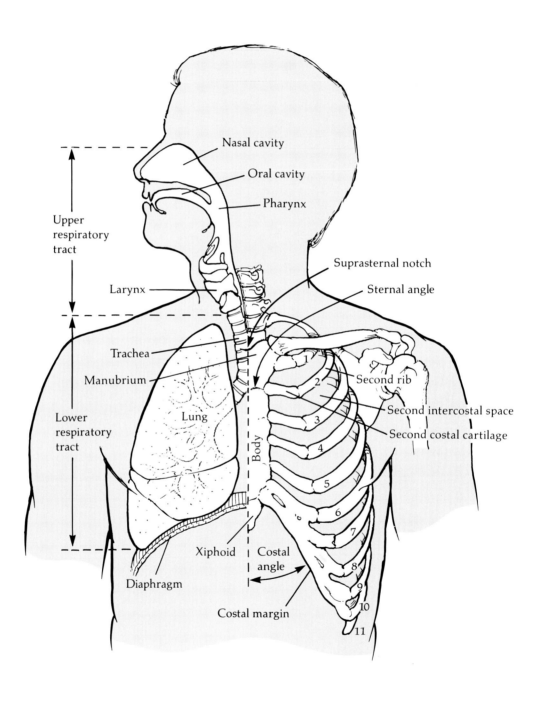

1.0   PULMONARY PHYSIOLOGY

The respiratory system has many functional characteristics that link both large and micro-scopic structures. The system consists of an upper airway, a lower airway, a bony or rigid thorax, the muscles of ventilation, a blood or perfusion system, and a control system (Figure 1.1). This system performs essential functions for the survival of the body, consisting of primary gas exchange as well as support of other body systems. These functions include:

Gas Exchange: The respiratory system supports all living cells in the body by providing a fresh supply of essential oxygen (O_2) for metabolism, and by removing carbon dioxide gas (CO_2), which is the waste product of metabolism.

Acid Base: Through the process of ventilation, the lung removes the appropriate amount of CO_2 gas and regulates the pH of the body. Regulation of pH is accomplished by removing volatile acid (acids converted into the gaseous state; in this case carbonic acid converted to CO_2 gas). At the same time, the kidneys regulate the fixed acids through the excretion of these acids in the urine.

Blood Reservoir: The lung receives the venous blood from the right ventricle of the heart. Because of its tremendous capacity to receive blood, the lung plays an essential role as the reservoir from which the left side of the heart draws blood.

Fluid Balance: The lung is capable of fluid absorption into the blood stream, as in the case of near drowning in fresh water or aspiration of fluids while drinking. The lung can also remove fluid from the blood stream, as in pulmonary edema during left ventricular failure.

Filtering Mechanism: The lung acts as a filtering mechanism for blood by removing several kinds of particles such as pulmonary emboli, fat emboli, bone marrow emboli, gas bubbles, and platelets or white cells. Filtered particles may be metabolized by the lung or removed through the lymphatics. The lung also constantly filters the air we breathe and removes trapped particles through the mucociliary clearance mechanism and the lymphatic system.

Temperature Control: Although humans use the lung only minimally as a cooling system, other species, such as dogs, depend heavily on the respiratory system to control body temperature.

Metabolism: The lung produces some very important chemicals that serve physiologic and regulatory functions such as: blood clotting, vascular dilation, lung structural stability, and neurotransmitters. Some chemicals passing through the lungs are converted into their more active form; for example, angiotensin I produced by the kidneys is converted to angiotensin II, a very potent vasoconstrictor.

Figure 1.2— Structure of the upper airway and the oral cavity.

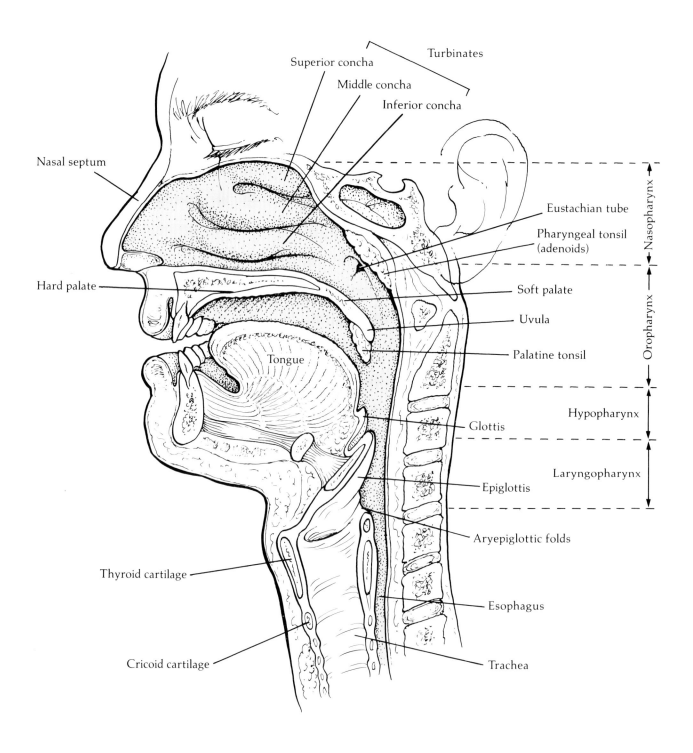

Turbinates

Superior concha

Middle concha

Inferior concha

Nasal septum

Eustachian tube

Pharyngeal tonsil (adenoids)

Nasopharynx

Hard palate

Soft palate

Uvula

Palatine tonsil

Tongue

Oropharynx

Glottis

Hypopharynx

Epiglottis

Laryngopharynx

Aryepiglottic folds

Thyroid cartilage

Esophagus

Cricoid cartilage

Trachea

1.1 *Upper Airway*

The upper airway acts as a conduction pathway for the movement of air into the respiratory system. Air passing through the upper airway is warmed, filtered, and humidified on its way to the respiratory exchange regions. The upper airway structures also function in speech and smell.

The upper airway includes the nose, the pharynx, and the larynx. Each of these structure has special functions (Figure 1.2).

The air "conditioning" process begins with the nose. Hair follicles in the anterior portion of the nose (the nares) help filter out large particles. The air then channels past three lateral bony plates called turbinates. Here, the air is exposed to mucous membranes that warm and humidify the gas. Irrespective of the coldness or dryness of inspired air, the gas is usually completely warmed to body temperature and saturated with water by the time it reaches the trachea. The mucous membranes contain goblet cells, which produce a mucous secretion, as well as tall columnar cells that contain cilia which help move the layer of mucous towards the throat. The mucous membranes are highly vascular and contribute about 650 milliliters of water to the inspired air per day. Large particles, greater than 10 microns in diameter, filter out in the nose while smaller particles, 2 to 10 microns in diameter, settle out in the mucociliary blanket of the lower respiratory tract.

The pharynx, the space behind the oral and nasal cavities, is subdivided into the nasopharynx, the oropharynx, and the laryngopharynx (Figure 1.2). The nasopharynx lies above the soft palate and contains the pharyngeal tonsils or adenoids. These structures consist of lymphatic tissue. If inflamed they can sometimes block off the eustachian tube that connects the throat to the middle ear.

The oropharynx includes the soft palate which spans the roof of the mouth to the base of the tongue. It functions as a conduit for air and food and contains the true tonsils (faucial tonsils) and the lingual tonsils, the lymph glands located at the base of the tongue.

The laryngopharynx is the section from the base of the tongue to the opening of the esophagus. It contains the glottis, the opening through which we breath, the epiglottis, and the aryepiglottic folds which cover and protect the airway during swallowing.

The larynx lies between the upper and lower airways and serves several important protective functions; it connects the upper and lower airways and is composed primarily of cartilage. Two large cartilage structures, the thyroid cartilage and the cricoid cartilage, form the structure for the voice box. Housed within this structure are the smaller arytenoid cartilages which are connected to the vocal cords. These cartilages, which move in response to very finely controlled musculature, are responsible for phonation. The epiglottis, located at the superior opening of the larynx, is an elastic cartilage attached to the thyroid cartilage. It closes over the opening of the airway during swallowing and protects the lower airway from aspiration of food particles or foreign bodies.

One of the more important functions of the larynx is the cough mechanism. Effective coughing clears particles from the larynx, trachea, and large airways. Clearance of particles that settle deeper in the airway depends on the mucociliary blanket described at the end of this section. The cough has several phases including irritation, deep inspiration, closure of the airway (glottic closure), compression and airway opening and expulsion. A cough can move gas from the lung at a rate of 10 liters per second during the expulsion phase.

Figure 1.3— Structure of the lower airway including the trachea, right and left main stem bronchi, and the lung segments originating form each of the segmental bronchi.

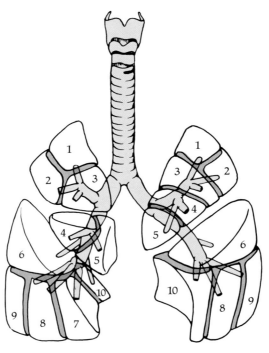

Figure 1.4— Airway branching in human lung by regularized dichotomy from trachea (generation Z=0) to alveolar ducts and sacs (generations 20 to 23).

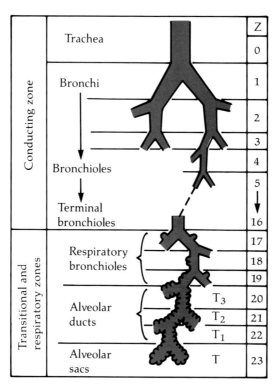

1.2 *Lower Airway*

1.2.1 Structural Considerations for the Lower Airway

The lower airway begins with the trachea and proceeds through some 25 generations of branching airways (Figures 1.3 and 1.4). The structural components of the airways coincide with their functional properties. The large airways contain cartilage that maintains airway patency, as well as large mucous glands and ciliated cells that support airway clearance. Smaller airways have bands of smooth muscle that help control the distribution of inspired air. Finally, tiny air sacs called alveoli are composed of very thin flat cells that form the network for gas exchange between fresh air containing air and venous blood.

On a macroscopic scale the lower airway consists of the trachea that bifurcates into two mainstem bronchi which conduct air to the right and left lungs. The mainstem bronchi branch consecutively to form three lobar bronchi on the right and two lobar bronchi on the left. Further branching results in 10 segmental bronchi on each side on the lung. This branching process continues, giving rise to three sequential groups of airways: the large or cartilaginous airways consisting of the trachea and the bronchi, the small airways or membranous airways called bronchioles, and the gas exchange region consisting of the respiratory bronchioles, alveolar ducts, and the alveoli.

1.2.2 Functional Considerations for the Lower Airway

The large cartilaginous airways, which function primarily in air conductance and filtration, include the trachea and the bronchi, generations 0 through 9. The bronchi, characterized by the cartilaginous layer, are embedded in the surrounding lung tissue (lung parenchyma), but are not directly connected to it. Their patency depends in part on their cartilaginous structure. In addition, the bronchial epithelium rests on spiral bands of smooth muscle whose tone depends on innervation from the autonomic nervous system and on chemical and humoral control. Even though the bronchi have relatively large diameters, the sum of their cross-sectional areas is small compared to the sum of the more distal airways. As a result, the large airways account for a larger portion of the resistance encountered when taking a breath.

Specialized cellular components, including the ciliated columnar cells, goblet cells, and submucosal glands, are adapted to support filtration and removal of foreign substances as well as maintaining airway humidification. Because of the thickness of these structural layers, the large airways receive their blood supply from a separate bronchial artery perfusion system.

The small airways consist of the bronchioles (generations 10 through 16) and are characterized by their bands of smooth muscle, lack of cartilage, and progressive decline in the number of goblet cells. In the bronchioles the clearance function diminishes and airway secretion becomes more serous. This design makes good sense because the airway size is now less than 2 millimeters in diameter. Because of the vast numbers of these small airways, their cross-sectional area is very large. Therefore, the bronchiolar conduction system contributes only about 10% of the total airway resistance during breathing. Small

Figure 1.5— Diagram of the functional respiratory unit, Acinus, consisting of one bronchiole, and its corresponding blood supply; pulmonary arteriole returning blood from the body, and pulmonary venule returning oxygenated blood from the alveoli to the left heart. The capillary network supplying the alveolus essentially forms a sheet of blood.

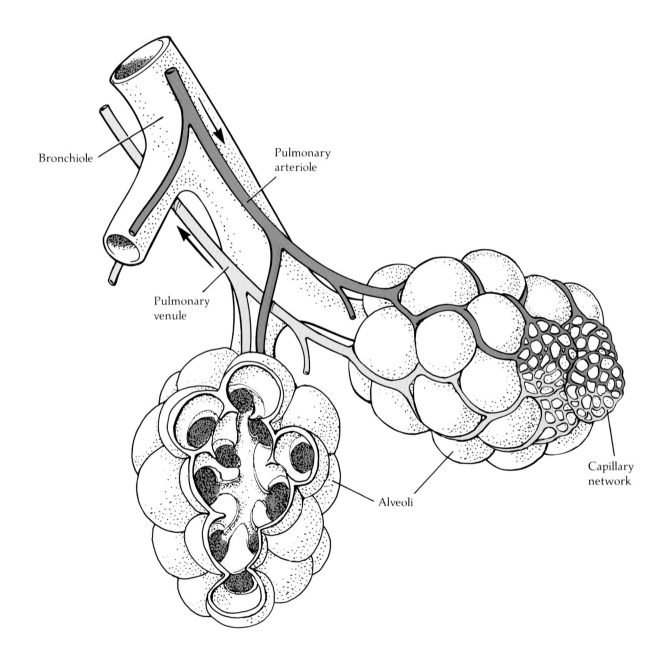

Bronchiole

Pulmonary arteriole

Pulmonary venule

Alveoli

Capillary network

changes in the caliber of these airways, however, have a tremendous effect on gas distribution to more distal lung units.

The transitional and respiratory zone begins with the respiratory bronchioles, the first region of gas exchange, and progresses to the alveoli (generations 17 through 23). The blood supply comes from the pulmonary circulation rather than the bronchial artery system. The gas exchange area does not contribute to airway resistance during breathing, but is involved in the distensibility, or compliance, of the lung.

The alveolar ducts arise from the respiratory bronchioles and act as conducting channels composed of alveoli separated by septal walls containing smooth muscle. Functionally, the ducts can contract or dilate in response to both humoral and chemical substances. Contraction or dilation affects lung distensibility. The alveolar ducts account for about 35% of the lungs' total gas exchange.

The final generation of the lung is the alveolus, the functional gas exchange unit. The acinus, or primary lobule, is a group of alveoli that form a functional respiratory unit supplying gas and blood for respiration. The acinus consists of approximately 3,000 alveoli. These alveoli receive fresh gas from one terminal bronchiole and blood from one pulmonary arteriole (not the bronchial artery). This functional gas exchange unit measures 3.5 millimeters in diameter, about the size of a pea (Figure 1.5). The lung contains about 100,000 acini and has a cross-sectional gas exchange area that approximates 75 square meters.

1.3 *Lung Clearance*

The lungs' protective mechanisms involve a combination of both mechanical and chemical means including filtration of inhaled particles in the nose and upper airway, coughing to remove large particles in the upper airway and major bronchi, tracheal bronchial clearance via the mucociliary blanket, bacterial clearance by alveolar macrophages and airway immunoglobulins, particulate removal through the lymphatic channels, and removal of solubilized substances by the bloodstream after passing through the alveolar capillary membrane. Particles are filtered by the respiratory system according to size.

The majority of trapped particles are removed from the lungs by the mucociliary blanket. The lungs produces approximately 100 milliliters of secretion each day. Cilia on the surface of the epithelial cells beat in a swaying motion to propel the mucous toward the larynx where it is eventually swallowed (Figure 1.6). This escalator mechanism moves the mucous about 1 to 2 centimeters per minute, approximately far enough to clear the lungs every hour.

Clinically, many respiratory diseases involve dysfunction of the mucociliary transport system. Chronic bronchitis, an example associated with increased mucous production, results from a proliferation of goblet cells and submucosal glands. In addition, several substances inhibit ciliary activity including alcohol, cigarette smoke, noxious gases, anesthetics, and low humidity.

Alveoli lie deep in the respiratory system below the areas containing cilia. They are located too distal in the lung for the cough mechanism to affect clearance. Clearance here relies on free-roaming alveolar macrophages and immunoglobulins. Macrophages contain enzymes that destroy bacteria, while immunoglobulins act as antibodies that fight bacteria and some viruses.

Figure 1.6— (a) The mucociliary escalator.
(b) Conceptual scheme of ciliary movement,
allowing forward motion to move viscous gel layer
and backward motion to take place entirely within
more fluid sol layer.

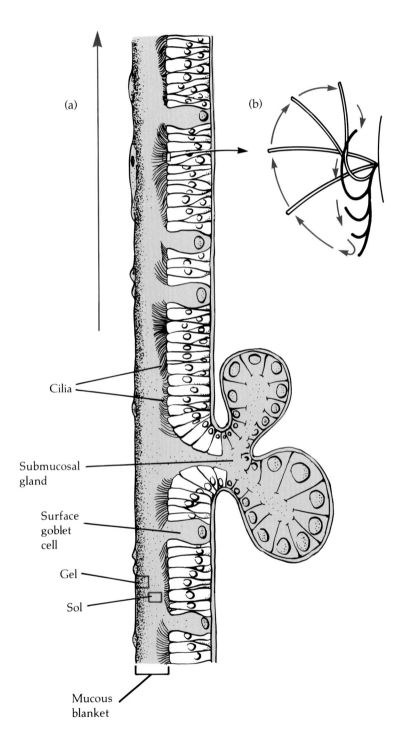

(a)

(b)

Cilia

Submucosal
gland

Surface
goblet
cell

Gel

Sol

Mucous
blanket

1.4   *Ventilation*

Ventilation, the movement of gas into and out of the lungs, requires an elastic lung and a flexible, expandable thoracic cage. The lungs act as pliable bellows that can hold up to six liters of gas and recoil to a volume of one liter after forced expiration. The thoracic cage is a three dimensional bone/cartilage structure serving as a rigid protector for the heart and lungs. The thorax is equipped with a complex system of muscles that expand in three dimensions — longitudinal, anterior-posterior, and transverse (lateral).

The thorax consists of 12 sets of paired ribs. Ten of the ribs are connected by cartilage to the sternum or the rib above. During the respiratory cycle, the cartilage attachments give the rib cage the flexibility required for expansion or contraction.

The muscles of ventilation are classified as primary or secondary according to their relative importance. The primary muscles include the diaphragm and two sets of intercostal muscles. The diaphragm elongates the thoracic cavity during inspiration and is innervated by the right and left phrenic nerves which originate from the spinal cord at the level of the third, fourth, and fifth cervical vertebrae. Damage to the spinal cord below this level leaves the diaphragm intact allowing the patient to continue to ventilate independently, while damage at or above this level results in diaphragmatic paralysis. The intercostal muscles consist of the external intercostals, which are primarily inspiratory muscles, and the internal intercostals, which assist the expiratory process.

The secondary muscles of ventilation include muscles of the neck, upper chest, back, and abdominals. Neck and upper chest muscles lift the upper ribs and sternum during inspiration, while the muscles of the chest and back act as accessory muscles of inspiration by elevating and helping to increase the diameter of the thoracic cage.

Abdominal muscles arise from portions of the lower eight ribs or their cartilages and are all expiratory muscles that function by compressing the abdominal space. This maneuver elevates the diaphragm as well as depressing the rib cage during forceful expiration. In addition, all of the abdominal muscles participate in coughing and sneezing.

1.5   *Static Lung Volumes*

Ventilation involves movement of air in and out of the chest. This process requires movement or changes in both the thoracic cage as well as the lung. Both systems are elastic in nature and stretch or compress according to the forces imposed by the ventilatory muscles. Before considering the dynamics of ventilation, however, it is important to understand how these two systems function at rest or during static conditions.

The lung and the thorax can be viewed as two elastic bands, each pulling in opposite directions on a pendulum (Figure 1.7). The lung is composed of elastic fibers and tends to recoil or collapse on its own. The thorax, on the other hand, consists of a group of ribs that have been pulled inward or bent by the elastic forces of the lungs. The normal tendency of the rib cage is to recoil in an outward direction. At rest, these two forces pull in equal but opposite directions and the imaginary pendulum rests in the middle. When muscular effort pulls the rib cage out, these forces are offset and the lung expands. When the muscles relax, the lung forces overpower the chest wall and exhalation occurs. Conversely, if muscular effort is used to compress the chest wall, the lung continues to exhale. Using the pendulum model as a framework, one can define normal tidal ventilation as well as static lung volumes and/or capacities (Figure 1.8).

Figure 1.7— Pendulum model of the lung illustrating the opposing forces of the lung and the chest wall.

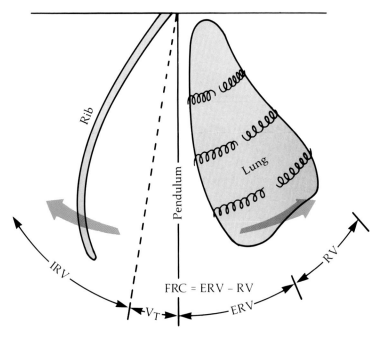

Figure 1.8— Spirograph illustrating lung volumes and capacities for a normal adult with a 6 liter total lung capacity (TLC). RV = residual volume, ERV = expiratory reserve volume, V_T = tidal volume, IRV = inspiratory reserve volume, FRC = functional residual capacity, IC = inspiratory capacity, VC = vital capacity.

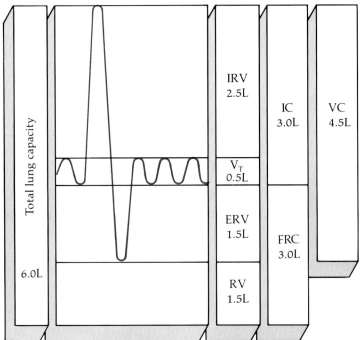

The amount of gas in the lung when the pendulum is at rest is called functional residual capacity (FRC). At this point, the lung elastic forces and the thoracic forces are equal but pulling in opposite directions. At rest, this volume of "functional" gas is exposed to the lung capillaries and constantly undergoes gas exchange.

Tidal volume (V_T) is the volume of gas moved during normal restful breathing. A small amount of muscular effort increases the size of the chest and expands the lung. Once the lung stretches, exhalation requires only that the muscles relax and the lung recoil naturally. The pendulum swings back and forth with each breath as a result of only a small muscular effort.

Expiratory reserve volume (ERV) is the amount of volume exhaled forcefully from the resting position. The pendulum is offset to the right as far as muscular effort can push it.

Residual volume (RV) is the amount of air remaining in the lung after a complete exhalation. The muscles of ventilation cannot completely collapse the thorax, leaving a certain amount of gas in the chest.

Inspiratory reserve volume (IRV) is the maximum amount of air that can be inhaled following a normal quiet inspiration. The muscles expand the thorax or move the pendulum as far left as possible.

1.6   *Measurement of Lung Volumes*

Lung volumes and ventilation are easily measured by a device called a spirometer. The spirometer consists of a breathing tube, a collection chamber (usually some sort of drum or cylinder), and a calibrated recording device. If the collection device is a cylinder, it is usually sealed by a rubber rolling seal that allows the cylinder to move without leaking any gas. A pen recording device, mechanically attached to the moving cylinder, records the volume movements as the cylinder moves during ventilation. The patient, usually seated in a chair, breathes normally at first then takes a deep breath to maximum lung capacity and performs a forced exhalation to residual volume. The resulting paper trace, called a spirograph, records each of the lung volumes (with the exception of the residual volume). Many modern spirometry systems convert this analog signal to digital analysis by computer, calculating accurately and quickly all the volumes and capacities described above. Section 2 reviews the common types of volume measuring devices and flow transducers used for the measurement of pulmonary function.

1.7   *Dynamic Ventilation*

The dynamics of ventilation involve a complex set of concepts including muscular movement that results in changes in the size and shape of the thorax and the lung, cyclic pressure changes in the thorax and lung resulting in gas movement and volume change, and gas distribution within the lung related to both compliance and resistance characteristics, normally referred to as lung mechanics.

Ventilation, frequently referred to as minute ventilation ($\dot{V}_E$), is the amount of gas moved in and out of the lung during a minute. Mathematically, it is the product of the tidal volume (V_T) and the breathing frequency (f):

$$\dot{V}_E = V_T \times f \qquad \textbf{Equation 1.1}$$

Figure 1.9— The tidal volume, (V_T) is a mixture of gas from the anatomical deadspace, (V_D) and from the alveolar gas, (V_A).

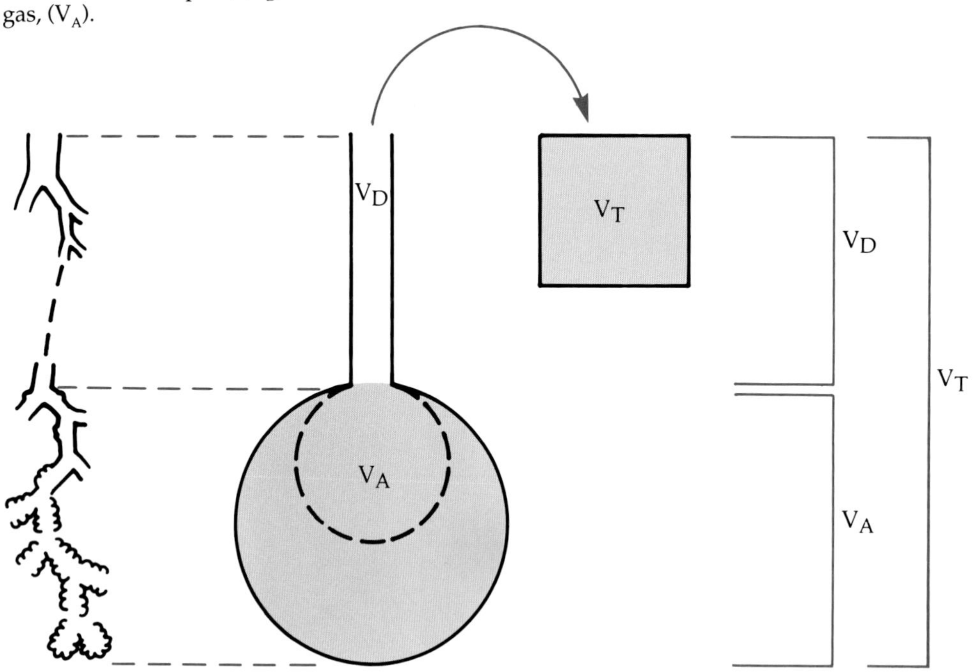

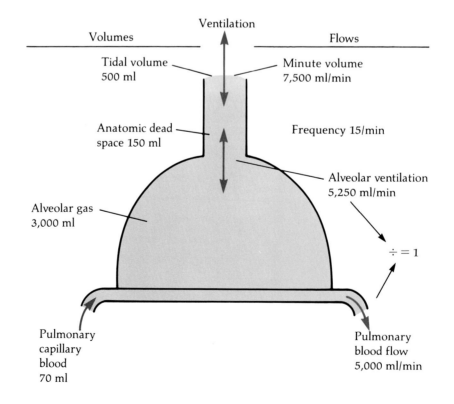

V_D

V_T

V_A

V_D

V_T

V_A

Figure 1.10— Diagram of a lung showing typical volumes and flows.

Volumes

Ventilation

Flows

Tidal volume
500 ml

Minute volume
7,500 ml/min

Anatomic dead
space 150 ml

Frequency 15/min

Alveolar ventilation
5,250 ml/min

Alveolar gas
3,000 ml

$\div = 1$

Pulmonary
capillary
blood
70 ml

Pulmonary
blood flow
5,000 ml/min

The amount of volume taken in during each breath (V_T) can be divided into two portions (Figure 1.9): alveolar gas volume (V_A), which undergoes gas exchange with alveolar capillaries, and deadspace gas (V_D), the amount of gas left in the conducting airways at the end of the breath or gas that reaches capillaries with no blood supply. This gas does not contribute to functional gas exchange:

$$V_T \;=\; V_A + V_D \qquad\qquad \text{Equation 1.2}$$

Deadspace gas may be further divided into:

■ Anatomic deadspace: primarily gas in the conducting airways.

■ Alveolar deadspace: alveoli not perfused and therefore not contributing to gas exchange.

■ Ventilation in excess of perfusion: alveoli over-ventilated in proportion to their perfusion and therefore having a portion of their ventilation functionally wasted.

■ Physiologic deadspace: the total amount of deadspace that exists; the sum of the three above representing the total amount of ventilation wasted or not physiologically effective.

Minute alveolar ventilation ($\dot{V}_A$), or minute deadspace ventilation ($\dot{V}_D$), may be derived by combining the two equations above (Figure 1.10):

$$
\begin{aligned}
\dot{V}_E \;&=\; (V_A + V_D) \times f \qquad\qquad \text{Equation 1.3}\\
&=\; (V_A \times f) + (V_D \times f)\\
&=\; \dot{V}_A + \dot{V}_D
\end{aligned}
$$

where
$$
\begin{aligned}
\dot{V}_E &= \text{minute ventilation}\\
V_A &= \text{alveolar gas volume}\\
V_D &= \text{deadspace gas}\\
f &= \text{breathing frequency.}
\end{aligned}
$$

Disease states can significantly alter the amount of deadspace ventilation, resulting in adverse effects on overall gas exchange. In addition, mechanical ventilators provide minute ventilation and must be adjusted to account for varying amounts of deadspace gas.

1.8 *Lung Mechanics*

The mechanical characteristics of the lung greatly influence both normal lung function and pulmonary disability. The two major factors involved in mechanics are lung compliance and resistance. Compliance generally refers to the static (no air flow) properties of the lung and measures the distensibility of the system when inflated with air. Resistance is a dynamic characteristic and is primarily concerned with the amount of pressure or work required to move air through the conducting pathways in the lung.

Ventilation is achieved by using muscles to alter the resting pressures within the thorax. Air can only move if pressure differences exist. Air moves from areas of higher pressure to areas of lower pressure. Thus, for air to move in and out of the lungs a pressure gradient must be created.

Normally, inspiration occurs when alveolar pressure falls below the atmospheric pressure. This negative pressure breathing uses the muscles of ventilation to decompress the gas in the chest, creating a less than ambient pressure. By contrast, positive pressure ventilation requires that a mechanism is used to compress air above ambient pressure.

Inspiration is normally accomplished by expansion of the thorax. As the diaphragm moves down and the chest wall moves outward, pressure surrounding the lung (intrapleural pressure) becomes more negative. This negative pressure decompresses the lung causing it to expand. As the lung expands, pressure inside the lung (alveolar pressure) drops below ambient pressure and air flows into the lung.

Unlike inspiration, which requires muscular effort, the expiratory process during the normal resting breathing pattern is mostly passive. As the inspiratory muscles relax, the lung's natural elastic fibers recoil. This recoil compresses lung volume and creates a positive alveolar pressure. As a result, a reverse gradient is created between the alveolar pressure and the atmosphere and the gas flows out of the lung.

1.9 *Static Property: Compliance*

The static characteristic of the lung, determined by its physical makeup, is called compliance. Lung expansion requires that the elastic forces which collapse the lung be stretched or overcome. To do this, the elastic and collagen fibers in the lung must be stretched, much like inflating a balloon. The stronger the elastic forces resisting inflation, the greater the pressure required to expand or to add volume to the lung. Elasticity is a measure of the force with which the lung fibers try to recoil. Compliance is the reciprocal of elasticity ($C = 1/E$), or a measure of how easily the lung distends. Compliance determines the volume change that will occur as a result of pressure changes imposed on the lung tissue. If the addition of volume to the lung requires only a small amount of pressure, the lung is called a compliant lung. On the other hand, if a large pressure is needed to inflate the lung, the lung is called a noncompliant lung. Compliance can be expressed as the relationship between volume and pressure or the volume change (ΔV) divided by the pressure change (ΔP):

$$\text{Compliance} = \frac{\text{Volume change } (\Delta V)}{\text{Pressure change } (\Delta P)} \qquad \textbf{Equation 1.4}$$

Mechanical ventilation of the lung involves expansion of the lung as well as the chest wall. Therefore, several kinds of compliance can be defined: lung compliance, chest wall compliance, and respiratory system or total compliance. Most ventilator systems are equipped to measure only respiratory system compliance. More recent monitoring equipment using esophageal balloons for measurement of pleural pressure can measure all three types of compliance.

Respiratory system compliance is measured by recording the tidal volume and the airway pressure during a mechanical breath. The laboratory tracing in Figure 1.11 represents a typical airway pressure record obtained during a series of tidal breaths. The inspiratory plateau can be created by dialing in the inspiratory pause on current ventilators. During inspiration, the peak pressure observed in the tracing is the pressure created in overcoming both resistance and compliance factors from the respiratory system and the ventilator circuit. During the plateau phase, however, airflow rapidly diminishes until the remaining pressure is predominantly produced by the elastic recoil properties of the system. The plateau pressure provides a reasonable estimate of the static recoil pressure resulting from the system's elasticity. Respiratory system compliance can then be calculated by dividing the tidal volume by the difference between plateau pressure and baseline pressure.

$$\text{Respiratory system compliance} = \frac{\text{Tidal volume}}{\text{Plateau pressure - Baseline pressure}} \qquad \textbf{Equation 1.5}$$

1.10   *Dynamic Property: Resistance*

In contrast to compliance, which is a measurement of the static properties of the pulmonary system, resistance refers to the dynamic flow-dependent properties of the lung-thorax system. Resistance to airflow within the system is calculated by the simultaneous measurement of airflow and the pressure required to produce the airflow. Pressure must be generated during breathing in order to overcome several kinds of resistance:

■ **Airway resistance:** Resistance specific to the movement of air through the conducting airways beginning with the mouth and/or nose and continuing all the way to the alveoli. For patients on mechanical ventilators, it includes the resistance of the ventilator circuitry and the endotracheal tube.

■ **Tissue viscous resistance:** The frictional resistance caused by movement of the tissues of the lung and the chest wall.

■ **Inertia:** Inertial forces must be applied to accelerate the gas and tissues that comprise the respiratory system. Physiologically, inertia has been found to be a negligible quantity during normal breathing.

Of the three types of resistance, airflow resistance is by far the most important clinically. The airflow resistance properties of the lung obey Poiseuille's law during conditions when the airflow is streamlined or laminar. Although turbulent flow also exists in the lung, the addition of turbulence does not alter the resistance of the airway per se, but rather changes the pressure required to produce the same amount of flow. Two major concepts from Poiseuille's law are clinically important: airway geometry and the pressure required to produce flow.

For Poiseuille's law:

$$\text{Flow} = \frac{(P_{in} - P_{out}) \pi r^4}{8 l n} \qquad \textbf{Equation 1.6}$$

where
$$P = \text{pressure}$$
$$r = \text{radius of tube (cm)}$$
$$n = \text{viscosity}$$
$$l = \text{length.}$$

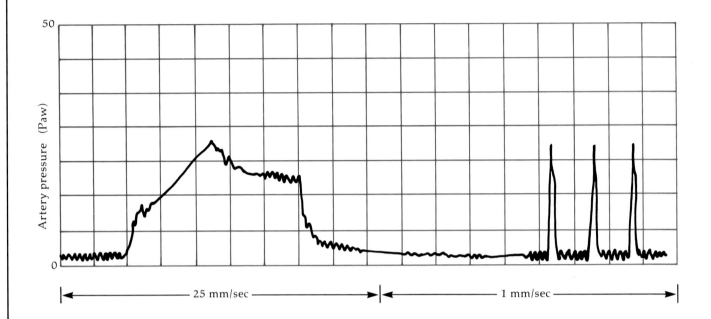

Figure 1.11— Airway pressure versus time graph from actual lung-ventilator trace.

50

Artery pressure (Paw)

0

|← ——— 25 mm/sec ——— →|← ——— 1 mm/sec ——— →|

Figure 1.12— Distribution of pleural pressure and transpulmonary pressure (lung distending pressure) in the upright lung. (a.) at rest and (b.) at the end of inspiration.

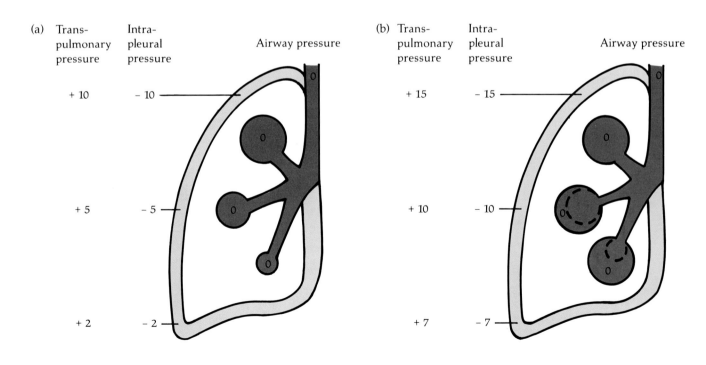

(a) Trans-pulmonary pressure | Intra-pleural pressure | Airway pressure

+ 10   − 10

+ 5   − 5

+ 2   − 2

(b) Trans-pulmonary pressure | Intra-pleural pressure | Airway pressure

+ 15   − 15

+ 10   − 10

+ 7   − 7

■ **Airway geometry**: Airflow resistance is primarily the result of the physical dimensions of the airway, with the radius being by far the most important factor. Lung pathologies related to resistance result from changes in radius; for example, bronchoconstriction, mucosal irritation and swelling, thickening of the mucosal layer, and airway compression. When the airway includes the endotracheal tube and ventilator circuitry, length as well as radius become important. In addition, water condensation in the tubing has a significant effect on the radius of the tubing and frequently becomes the largest resistance factor in the circuit.

■ The pressure required to achieve a constant flow changes every time the airway geometry changes. Disease states that reduce the radius of the airways require increased amounts of pressure to produce airflow. As a consequence, the patient must work harder to breathe.

Although it is possible to measure several different kinds of resistance, this section will discuss only total system resistance, including the resistance of the lung, the chest wall, and portions of the ventilator circuit. Resistance can be calculated from the general equation:

$$\text{Resistance} \ = \ \frac{\text{Pressure difference}}{\text{Flow}} \qquad \textbf{Equation 1.7}$$

where   Pressure difference = difference between peak pressure and plateau pressure

                   Flow = airflow.

From Figure 1.11, resistance can be determined by dividing the difference between peak pressure and plateau pressure by airflow. Since plateau pressure represents the elastic forces of the system, one can assume that the remaining pressure difference $(P_1 - P_2)$ is the pressure required to overcome the resistance of the system at the moment airflow stops. Airflow values may be obtained from specific airflow-sensing devices located on the mechanical ventilator or on airway monitoring instruments. On ventilators not equipped with these devices, airflow may be approximated by recording the flow setting on the ventilator, provided the ventilator generates a square wave or constant flow pattern. Resistance measurements from ventilators producing sine wave or diminishing flow patterns are less accurate, but still indicate the direction in which resistance changes occur in the patient's respiratory system.

1.11 *Distribution of Volume and Ventilation*

Two important consequences of the mechanical properties of the lung are the distribution of volume and the distribution of ventilation. The distribution of volume in the upright lung is determined by two factors: the inflation curve or volume pressure curve for the lung, where the shape of this curve is entirely determined by the compliance of the lung and the effect of gravity on the lung.

The lung inflation curve can be determined by inflating the lung in stepwise increments and simultaneously measuring the amount of pressure required to achieve inflation. Figure 1.12 illustrates that the lung inflates in a curved or "S" shaped pattern. This

Figure 1.13— Effect of regional differences in pleural pressure on the distribution of ventilation.

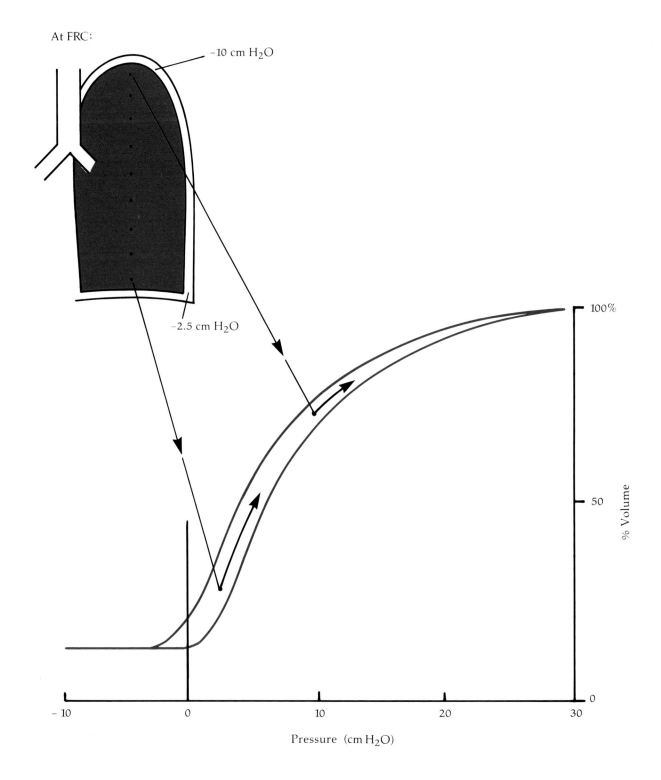

At FRC:

-10 cm H$_2$O

-2.5 cm H$_2$O

100%

50

% Volume

0

-10   0   10   20   30

Pressure (cm H$_2$O)

pattern results from the elastic nature of the lung and surface tension characteristics. The amount of volume in any given unit is determined by the amount of inflating pressure or transpulmonary pressure to which the lung unit is exposed, and the lung elasticity.

At rest or at the end of a tidal exhalation, the lung units experience different transpulmonary pressures or different distending pressures as a result of the effect of gravity on the lung. The lung has considerable weight due to the volume of blood filling the capillaries. Therefore, the distending pressures are less in the bottom of the lung than at the top. As a result, in the upright resting position, the apical lung units expand more than the basilar units (Figure 1.13).

The distribution of ventilation during tidal breathing is opposite to distribution of volume that occurs at rest. In the upright position the lower lung units receive more ventilation than the upper lung units. Ventilation, a dynamic process, refers to the amount of volume change that occurs during a breath. The amount of ventilation that a lung unit receives is determined by the lung unit's initial location on the lung volume pressure curve before the breath starts and on the amount of additional distending pressure that the unit is exposed to. If two lung units are exposed to the same change in pressure during a breath, the amount of inflation depends on their respective initial location on the inflation curve. Generally, the basal units are located at the beginning of the steep portion of the inflation curve, while the apical units remain near the top or flat portion of the inflation curve. As shown in Figure 1.13, the basal units move a considerable distance up the curve during the breath and have a large resultant volume change or ventilation. The apical units, which initially have a large resting volume, have a relatively small volume change during the breath. The larger ventilation in the basal units in the upright lung is beneficial because, proportionately, more blood flow is also distributed to this region.

1.12 *Gas Exchange*

The exchange of O_2 used for metabolism or CO_2 produced by the metabolic process occurs across the alveolar capillary membrane. This exchange process is influenced by a number of physical factors including the solubility of the diffusing gases and their reactions with the blood, the properties of the alveolar capillary membrane across which the diffusion process must occur, the supply of fresh gas, the supply of blood, and the matching of ventilation with perfusion or the ventilation/perfusion ratio.

Gas exchange takes place at two different levels in the body: externally in the lung and internally through the tissue capillaries that supply O_2 directly to tissue cells (Figure 1.14).

External gas exchange, or external respiration, refers to exchange that occurs at the alveolar capillary level in the lung. This exchange between O_2 supplied from the atmosphere by ventilation and venous blood supplied to the lung capillaries is controlled by two systems: a ventilation system and a blood flow system. These systems, which control or determine external gas exchange, must be able to meet the metabolic needs of the cells lying deep within the organism in order for the organism to survive.

Internal respiration refers to the gas exchange occurring between the systemic capillary and the actual tissue cells. The need for O_2 and removal of CO_2 at this level is entirely dependent on the metabolic activity of the cell. For the organism to live, the gas exchange needs of the cells (internal respiration) must be balanced by the external gas exchange mechanism.

Figure 1.14— Gas exchange (respiration) takes place both internally and externally in the body.

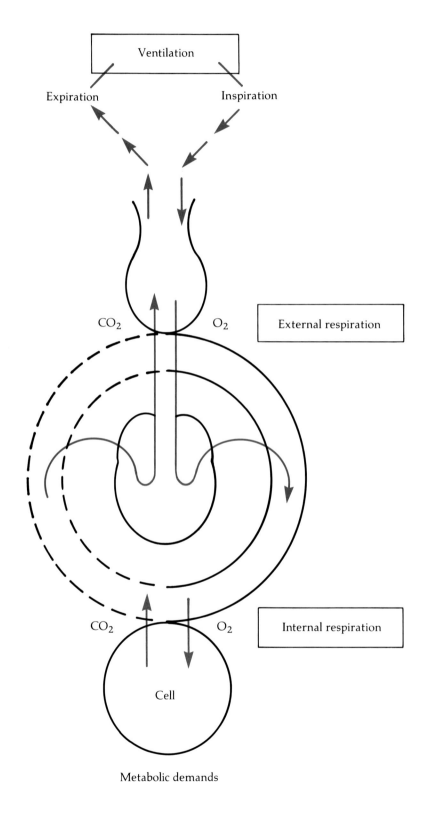

Four primary factors influence the external gas exchange process:

- **Ventilation**: Gases must move in and out of the respiratory system. This involves the use of the ventilatory muscles and a ventilatory control system.

- **Diffusion**: Gases move across membranes and into and out of cells because of their tendency to move from areas of higher kinetic energy to areas of lower kinetic energy or concentration.

- **Perfusion**: Blood flows through the lung and specifically through the pulmonary capillaries. Blood flow facilitates the diffusion process and is the essential carrier mechanism for transport of gases to and away from the tissue cells.

- **Ventilation perfusion ratio**: This ratio determines the amounts of O_2 and CO_2 exchanged in each lung unit. By very carefully controlling this ratio, the body can match the external gas exchange process to the internal cellular needs.

External respiration depends on the ventilation perfusion ratio. Gas exchange between the atmosphere and the blood results from the gas exchange between individual alveolar air units and the pulmonary blood perfusing the alveolar capillary. This combination of alveolus and corresponding pulmonary capillary forms the basic respiratory unit (Figure 1.15).

It is helpful to consider the respiratory unit in terms of the amount of ventilation relative to the amount of perfusion. In fact, an infinite number of variations occur between the two ends of the spectrum, from completely ventilated but not perfused to completely perfused but not ventilated. The variations can be simplified as follows:

- **Normal unit:** The normal respiratory unit is both ventilated and perfused. Venous blood returning from the tissue cells is exposed to fresh alveolar gas and exits the capillary replenished with O_2.

- **Deadspace unit:** This respiratory unit is ventilated but not perfused. From a gas exchange standpoint, this is wasted ventilation.

- **Shunt unit:** This respiratory unit represents a pulmonary capillary that is perfused but not ventilated. The blood in this capillary bypasses the gas exchange process and lowers the O_2 tension in the arterial blood.

- **Silent unit:** This respiratory unit is neither ventilated nor perfused.

1.13 *Diffusion*

Diffusion across membranes and through tissues is described by Fick's law. This law states that the rate of diffusion ($\dot{V}$) of a gas across a membrane is proportional to the surface area of the membrane (A), a diffusion coefficient (D), the partial pressure differences or concentration difference between the two sides of the membrane (P_1-P_2), and inversely proportional to the thickness of the membrane (t):

Figure 1.15— Basic respiratory unit: ventilated alveolus and corresponding pulmonary capillary. Gas exchange is the net result of fresh air exchange in the alveolus in relation to mixed venous blood supply. Normal values for carbon dioxide tension are illustrated.

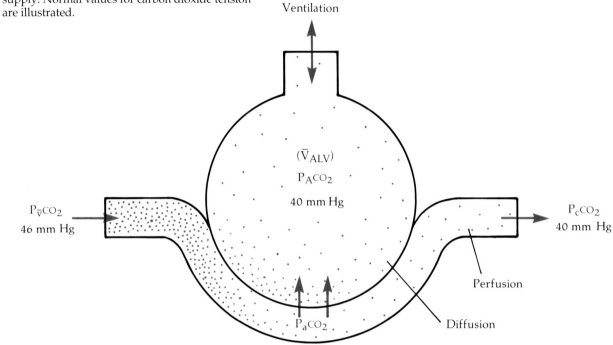

Figure 1.16— Diffusion cascade: schematic representation of the partial pressures of O_2 and CO_2 as they change from the atmosphere to the tissue cells.

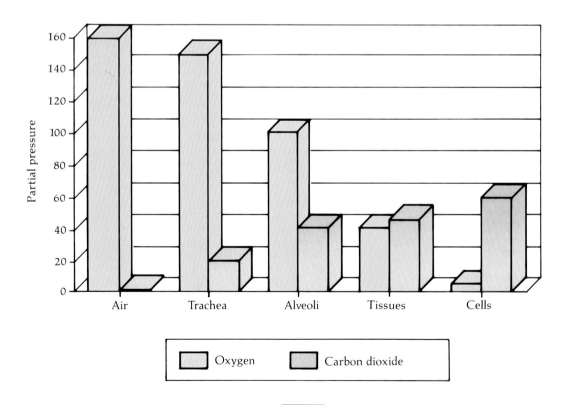

$$\dot{V} = \frac{A\,D\,(P_1 - P_2)}{t}$$

Equation 1.8

where

$\dot{V}$ = rate of diffusion
A = surface area of the membrane
D = diffusion coefficient
$P_1 - P_2$ = partial pressure differences across the membrane
t = thickness of the membrane.

Although certain disease states affect these variables (for example, emphysema and pneumonectomy affect surface area; pulmonary edema and fibrosis affect membrane thickness), the main focus here will be on the pressure gradients that move gases within the system.

Oxygen flows or moves down pressure gradients beginning with the partial pressure of O_2 in the inspired air and ending in the partial pressure of the mitochondria within the tissue cells. Pictorially, this is often represented as the O_2 cascade (Figure 1.16). Oxygen enters the respiratory system at a P_aO_2 of approximately 160 mm Hg. A slight drop in pressure results from the addition of humidity in the upper airway, followed by a large drop as the inspired air mixes with the large amount of functional residual volume that exists in the lung during normal breathing. Diffusion occurs across the alveolar capillary membrane as pressure gradients move the O_2 into the alveolar capillary blood. Oxygen-rich arterial blood is then pumped to the tissue capillaries where pressure-driven diffusion again occurs between the blood and the tissue cells. Finally, O_2 further diffuses within the tissue and into the interior of each cell where the mitochondria use it for cellular metabolism.

The movement of O_2 across the alveolar capillary membrane depends on the pressure differences between the alveolar gas and the capillary blood. Normally the alveolar gas has a partial pressure of approximately 100 mm Hg while the mixed venous blood has a partial pressure of 40 mm Hg. Thus, the initial pressure gradient moving O_2 into the blood is approximately 60 mm Hg. As the diffusion process continues to occur, this pressure gradient gradually diminishes until the capillary blood has equilibrated with the alveolar gas. Figure 1.17 presents the time course of this process. Pulmonary blood requires only about one third of this time to equilibrate with the alveolar gas. As a result, the normal lung has a fairly large diffusion reserve. Normally, movement of O_2 is not limited by the diffusion process but rather by the amount of blood perfusing the capillary. Since the O_2 concentration equilibrates so rapidly across the membrane, the factor that limits the amount of O_2 diffusing across the membrane is the amount of pulmonary blood flow.

1.14 *Pulmonary Blood Flow*

The gas exchange process requires both ventilation and pulmonary blood flow. Blood flow is essential in achieving O_2 uptake in the lungs as well as in delivering CO_2 from the tissue to the lungs. The lungs receive the entire cardiac output from the right heart. The pulmonary perfusion system consists of a branching network of pulmonary arteries that distribute venous blood to the alveolar capillaries for gas exchange. In addition, a second and much smaller perfusion system exists — the bronchial artery system. This system supplies oxygenated systemic blood to the walls of the tracheal bronchial tree. The additional blood supply is necessary because of the metabolic activity required to support the

Figure 1.17— Diffusion profile for O_2 and CO_2.
Mixed venous blood enters the capillary on the left
and begins to equilibrate with alveolar gas tension
(dashed lines).

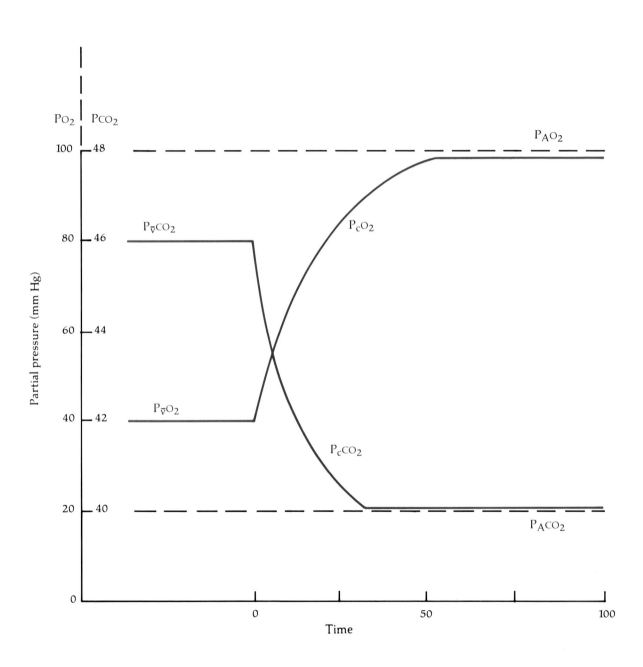

mucociliary transport system and because the bronchial walls are too thick to receive O_2 via diffusion from the airway.

1.15   *Pulmonary Circulation*

The lung is perfused by two main pulmonary arteries, one entering from the left and the other from the right, close to the middle, or hilum, of the lung. Each of these arteries branch along with their respective bronchi, becoming smaller and smaller until they eventually form a sheet-like capillary network called the alveolar capillary. This extremely thin (1 to 2 microns) capillary network facilitates the diffusion process. For the most part blood flows through the capillary as a single layer or sheet of red cells.

Structurally, pulmonary arteries contain less smooth muscle than systemic arteries. The thin wall structures result in a much more distensible vessel, a characteristic that not only allows the pulmonary arteries to stretch with lung inflation but also permits them to function as a blood reservoir for the heart.

1.16   *Pulmonary Vascular Pressures and Resistance*

Pressures in pulmonary circulation are much smaller than pressures in the systemic system. Pulmonary artery pressure measures approximately 25/8 mm Hg with a mean of 15 mm Hg, compared to a normal systemic arterial blood pressure of 120/80 mm Hg and a mean of 100 mm Hg. The structural differences in the pulmonary arterial walls described above and their increased distensibility contribute to decreased blood pressure. Because of the smaller pressures in the pulmonary circulation, resistance is only one tenth that of the systemic system.

Lung perfusion pressure as well as lung inflation affect pulmonary vascular resistance. Increased perfusion pressure decreases vascular resistance as a result of recruitment of additional pulmonary vessels (probably in the apex of the lung) and distension of other vessels. In addition, lung inflation has a variable effect on resistance as illustrated in Figure 1.18. Pulmonary vascular resistance increases as the lung deflates below FRC as well as when the lung volume increases above FRC. This results from the varying effect that lung volume has on the pulmonary vessels according to location. Vessels course along with branching airways until they become alveolar capillary vessels. Before they reach the capillary, however, they branch with the airways and embed in the lung parenchyma (lung tissue). Before joining the capillary these vessels are surrounded by alveoli and are called extra alveolar vessels. During lung inflation, the alveoli stretch and exert radial tension on the extra alveolar vessels causing them to dilate.

In contrast, once the pulmonary vessels reach the capillary, they become part of the alveolar wall. Lung inflation in this instance stretches the wall and narrows the alveolar vessel. As illustrated in Figure 1.18, the lowest vascular resistance occurs at functional residual volume, the volume where the lung spends the majority of its time.

1.17   *Distribution of Pulmonary Blood Flow*

Blood flow is unevenly distributed in the lung as a result of two primary factors: the available perfusion pressure created by the right heart, and the affect of gravity on the lung. Figure 1.19 illustrates the three zones of lung perfusion.

Figure 1.18— The effects of lung volume on pulmonary vascular resistance.

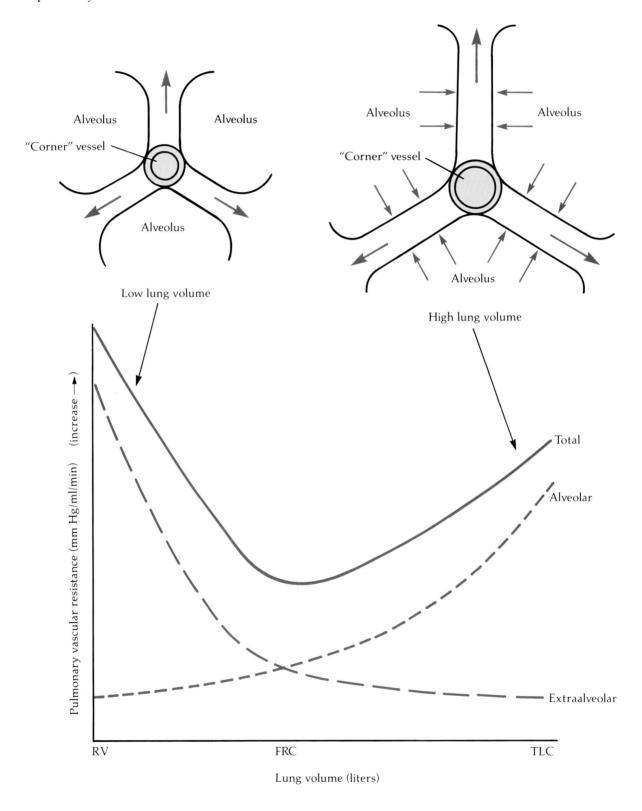

Figure 1.19— Scheme which accounts for the distribution of blood flow in the isolated lung.

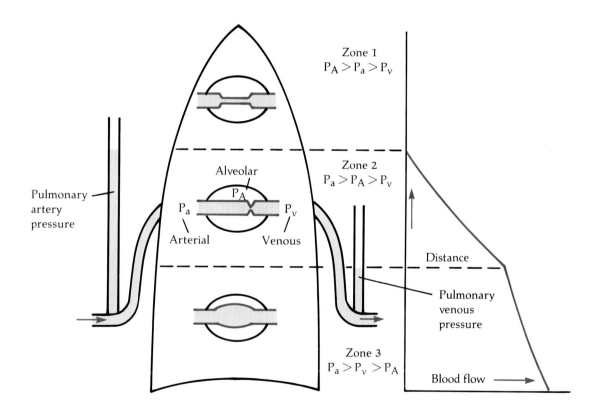

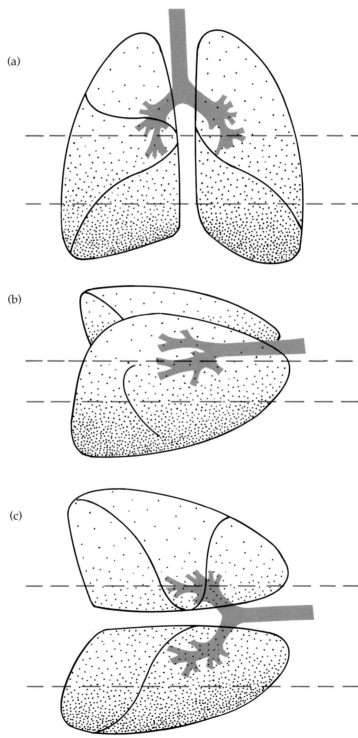

Figure 1.20— The majority of pulmonary blood flow normally occurs in the gravity-dependent areas of the lung. Thus, body position has a significant effect on the distribution of pulmonary blood flow, as shown in the erect (a), supine (lying on the back) (b), and lateral (lying on the side) (c) positions.

In zone 1 no blood flow occurs because the pulmonary perfusion pressure is not sufficient to pump blood to this level. For the most part, normal individuals do not have a zone 1. However, it tends to appear in very tall persons or during conditions of positive pressure, such as during intermittent positive pressure breathing (IPPB) or mechanical ventilation where the alveolar pressure causes the capillary to collapse.

Blood flow increases in zone 2. This zone resembles a vessel within an airtight box. Blood flow in this region depends on both the arterial perfusion pressure and the alveolar pressure. The arterial pressure supports blood flow through the vessel, but the flow can be reduced by increasing the air pressure inside the box. The amount of blood flow depends on the difference between the arterial perfusion pressure and the air or alveolar pressure. The flow in this zone may be described as the waterfall effect or the *Starling Resistor Phenomenon*, where the alveolar pressure represents the dam (the blood flow downstream of the dam is controlled by the dam).

Blood flow is greatest in zone 3 where the perfusion pressure always exceeds the alveolar pressure. Blood flow occurs as a result of the difference between pulmonary artery pressure and pulmonary venous pressure. This pressure difference is constant throughout the zone. Blood flow increases deeper into the zone, however, because the mean pressure within the vessel increases and distends the vessel.

These three zones are constantly shifting as body position changes. As seen in Figure 1.20, gravity has the effect of retaining the vertical orientation such that the uppermost lung section becomes the new zone 1 and the lowermost lung section becomes zone 3. The lung is most evenly perfused in the recumbent position where a larger percentage of the total lung exists as zone 3.

1.18 *Ventilation Perfusion Relationships*

The relationship between ventilation and perfusion affects the gas exchange process. Even distribution or equal matching of ventilation and perfusion maximizes gas exchange, while imbalance between the two impairs gas exchange. The pathology of most lung disorders results from ventilation/perfusion mismatch.

1.18.1 Impaired Gas Exchange

Gas exchange is often compared to heat exchange in a hot water heater. The efficiency of the heat exchange device can be determined by measuring how closely the air temperature coming out of the device matches the temperature of the water inside the device. If the difference is large, the device is not a very good heat exchanger. Similarly, the ability of the lung to exchange gas can be measured by determining how closely the O_2 tensions in the arterial blood (blood returning from the lung after the gas exchange process, P_aO_2) match the O_2 tension inside the lung (the alveolar P_AO_2). Under perfect conditions, the P_aO_2 and P_aCO_2 would exactly match the corresponding P_AO_2 and P_ACO_2. During normal conditions, however, a small difference exists between the arterial and alveolar gas concentrations (usually less than 5 mm Hg for O_2). This difference can become significantly larger and the gas exchange process can become significantly impaired as a result of any of the four following conditions: hypoventilation, diffusion impairment, shunting of blood, and ventilation/perfusion inequality.

Figure 1.21— Extremes of ventilation-perfusion ratio.

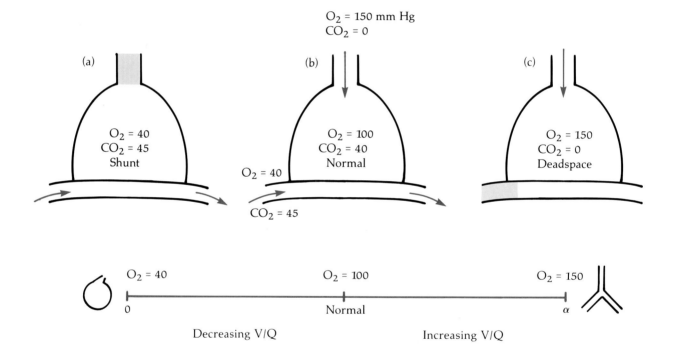

O_2 = 150 mm Hg
CO_2 = 0

(a)

O_2 = 40
CO_2 = 45
Shunt

(b)

O_2 = 40

O_2 = 100
CO_2 = 40
Normal

CO_2 = 45

(c)

O_2 = 150
CO_2 = 0
Deadspace

O_2 = 40

O_2 = 100

O_2 = 150

0

Normal

α

Decreasing V/Q

Increasing V/Q

Hypoventilation: The P_AO_2 is determined by comparing the rate of removal of O_2 by the blood and the rate of replenishment by alveolar ventilation. Hypoventilation has two negative effects on the gas exchange process. First, fresh O_2 is not replenished in the lung so that the arterial O_2 tensions begin to approach those of venous blood. Second, as the alveolar gas tensions drop, the partial pressure gradient between gas and blood diminishes. This gradient is necessary for the gases to move across the capillary membrane.

Diffusion Impairment: Actual diffusion impairment occurs under conditions in which the alveolar capillary membrane becomes thickened, such as in pulmonary edema. In addition, exercise and altitude affect the diffusion capabilities of the lung by reducing the time that gas has to diffuse across the membrane and the partial pressure gradient that drives diffusion. Although diffusion impairment can and does occur in the clinical setting, the primary gas exchange limitation usually results from ventilation perfusion inequality.

Shunt: Shunted blood never exchanges with alveolar gas and, therefore, has the immediate effect of lowering the arterial O_2 tension below the alveolar level. Because true shunted blood is not exposed to the alveolar gas, supplemental O_2 is of little use in correcting the gas exchange problem. However, in lung units with very small amounts of ventilation and normal perfusion (called the shunt effect or perfusion in excess of ventilation), the use of supplemental O_2 is quite beneficial. The additional O_2 increases the partial pressure of the gas in the alveolus and, therefore, supports the diffusion process.

Ventilation/Perfusion: The inequality of ventilation and perfusion is the most common cause of impaired gas exchange in the lung. Even though the normal amount of inequality in gas pressures makes surprisingly little difference (only 5 mm Hg for O_2 and only about 1 mm Hg for CO_2), in disease states the mismatch accounts for very large and critical differences. For example, consider how the gas exchange function of the lung would be impaired if all ventilation went to the apex of the lung and all perfusion went to the base of the lung. Gas exchange would not occur at all because fresh gas would never come in contact with capillary blood. While this is an extreme case, and the lung as a whole does not usually exhibit this tendency, certain disease states occur in which many sections of the lung have widely varying degrees of ventilation and blood flow.

1.18.2 Ventilation Perfusion Ratio

It is helpful when considering the relationship between ventilation and perfusion to look at the ventilation/perfusion (V/Q) line (Figure 1.21). This line expresses the extremes of V/Q that may occur in the lung and the range of gas tensions that occur as a result of this relationship. The V/Q line begins with a lung unit that has no ventilation, for example, a shunt unit that has a V/Q ratio of 0. It proceeds through the normal ventilation perfusion ratio of about 0.8 to 1 and finally increases until an infinite amount of ventilation exists compared to blood flow, namely, deadspace.

The normal condition of the lung is near the middle of the V/Q line, with the bases lying slightly to the left and the apices slightly to the right. As described earlier, the bases of the lung are more heavily perfused than the apices and have a lower V/Q ratio. By contrast, the apices have a relatively small amount of perfusion and are comparatively over-ventilated relative to their perfusion. This relationship can be expressed as a chart illustrating the ventilation perfusion rations for different cross-sections of the lung from the

Figure 1.22— Regional differences in gas exchange down the normal lung. Only the apical and basal values are shown.

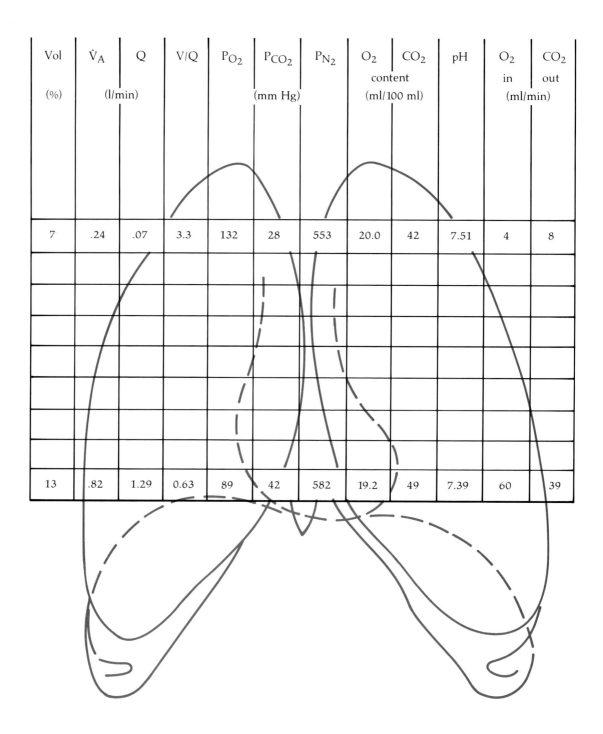

Vol	$\dot{V}_A$	Q	V/Q	P_{O_2}	P_{CO_2}	P_{N_2}	O_2 content	CO_2	pH	O_2 in	CO_2 out
(%)	(l/min)				(mm Hg)		(ml/100 ml)			(ml/min)	
7	.24	.07	3.3	132	28	553	20.0	42	7.51	4	8
13	.82	1.29	0.63	89	42	582	19.2	49	7.39	60	39

base to the apex (Figure 1.22). In this chart, the apex has a ventilation perfusion ratio of about 3.3 and the base has a V/Q = 0.6.

The importance of the ventilation perfusion ratio in determining gas exchange can also be described by considering the O_2-CO_2 diagram (Figure 1.23). This diagram illustrates the alveolar gas tensions and blood tensions resulting from all the possible combinations of ventilation and blood flow or all the V/Q ratios. Each lung slice is represented on the graph by a point. Lung slices near the apex appear far to the right and more closely resemble that of deadspace or inspired gas tensions. Lung units to the left represent units from the base of the lung with lower V/Q ratios and more closely approximate shunt or mixed venous blood.

1.19   *Gas Transport*

For multiple-celled organisms to survive in the evolutionary process, they had to develop systems that would effectively transport gases (O_2) from the external environment internally to individual cells. As a benefit to the organism, the transition from anaerobic life to aerobic life allowed for 18 times as much energy to be extracted from metabolism of glucose in the presence of O_2. Two principal mechanisms evolved for providing a continuous flow of O_2 to the cells: a circulatory system (because O_2 has a diffusion limitation of about 1 millimeter in tissue), and O_2-carrying molecules (proteins) capable of greatly increasing the amount of O_2 transported by the blood. Functionally, O_2 must be transported to the cells for metabolism and CO_2 must be transported away from the cells and removed from the body. Because transport of these gases requires significantly different mechanisms, they will be discussed separately.

1.19.1 Oxygen Transport

Blood carries O_2 in two forms: dissolved in the plasma and attached or bound to hemoglobin. Oxygen content refers to the sum of both forms contained in a blood sample and is usually reported in volumes percent (vol%) or the amount of O_2 in milliliters that is contained in 100 milliliters of blood. Normally about 20 vol%, or 20 milliliters of O_2, are carried in every 100 milliliters of arterial blood.

The amount of O_2 dissolved in plasma is a function of the solubility of O_2 in plasma and the partial pressure of O_2 in the sample. The solubility is determined chemically and is generally reported as 0.003 vol% or, for every 100 milliliters of blood, 0.003 milliliters of O_2 per mm Hg of O_2 tension.

The vast majority of O_2 molecules in the blood are bound to hemoglobin molecules within the red blood cells. Hemoglobin, a very large protein molecule with a molecular weight of 64,457 grams, consists of four large protein portions (four globins) and four heme groups (a nonprotein portion containing iron). Oxygen is carried or bound by the iron portion of the heme group. Each molecule of hemoglobin has four iron sites and can carry four O_2 molecules. The presence of hemoglobin in the blood increases the O_2 transport capabilities of one liter of blood from about 3 milliliters to 200 milliliters of O_2.

Oxygen combines with hemoglobin in an easily reversible reaction to form oxyhemoglobin. The binding process, however, is affected by the number of O_2 molecules already bound to the hemoglobin molecule and by several other important factors that affect the binding capability including the presence of CO_2 and hydrogen ions (which are also carried by hemoglobin), temperature, and 2,3-diphosphoglycerate. Increases in the

Figure 1.23— Oxygen-carbon dioxide diagram.

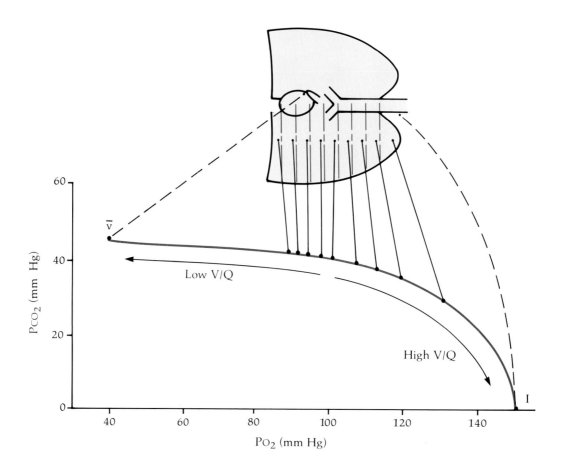

concentration of CO_2, hydrogen ions, and 2,3-diphosphoglycerate, or an increase in the temperature alter the binding characteristics of hemoglobin, resulting in O_2 release. This process occurs at the tissue level where O_2 is unloaded to the cells. Conversely, decreases in these same factors increase the affinity of the hemoglobin molecule for O_2 as it passes through the lung and, therefore, assist the loading of O_2 onto the red blood cell.

The binding of O_2 to hemoglobin is expressed as the oxyhemoglobin curve (Figure 1.24). The sigmoid shape of this curve reflects the change in binding characteristics of hemoglobin as the four O_2 molecules are added on to the hemoglobin. In addition, by expressing the vertical axis as O_2 content, one can see the differences in the amounts of O_2 carried as dissolved versus that bound to hemoglobin. One gram of pure hemoglobin when fully saturated with O_2 combines with 1.39 milliliters of O_2. Under normal body conditions, which include small amounts of impurities, this value is reduced to 1.34 milliliters of O_2 and is the standard value reported in most textbooks.

The total amount of O_2 carried by a 100-milliliter sample of arterial blood is the sum of the O_2 bound to hemoglobin and that which is dissolved in the plasma:

- Bound O_2: 15 gm%Hb x 1.34 mls/gm x 98% saturation = 19.69 vol%

- Dissolved O_2: .003 vol% x 100 mm Hg P_{O_2} = 00.3 vol%

Total O_2 = 19.99 vol%

where Hb = hemoglobin

P_{O_2} = partial pressure of O_2
mm Hg = millimeters of mercury pressure.

For cells to use O_2 in metabolism, the O_2 must be transported from the lung to the tissue. The heart moves the O_2 using the hemoglobin of the red blood cell as the primary gas transport medium. The total amount of O_2 transported to the tissues by the arterial blood can be calculated by multiplying the cardiac output times the blood O_2 content:

$$O_2 \text{ transport } = \text{ Cardiac output } x O_2 \text{ content} \qquad \textbf{Equation 1.9}$$

Since O_2 content is expressed in volumes percent or the number of milliliters of O_2 contained in 100 milliliters of blood, the cardiac output must be converted into the number of 100-milliliter units delivered per minute. Cardiac output is reported as liters per minute so the conversion is accomplished by multiplying the cardiac output by 10:

$$O_2 \text{ transport } = \text{ (CO x 10) x } C_aO_2 \qquad \textbf{Equation 1.10}$$

where CO = cardiac output
C_aO_2 = O_2 content of arterial blood.

1.19.2 Carbon Dioxide Transport

Carbon dioxide originates as a byproduct of metabolism in the cells. It diffuses out of the cells and into the capillary venous blood where it is carried to the lungs for elimination. Carbon dioxide is carried in two primary compartments: in the plasma and within the red blood cells. In contrast to O_2, which is transported primarily bound to hemoglobin, much

Figure 1.24— Oxygen content and hemoglobin saturation diagrams.

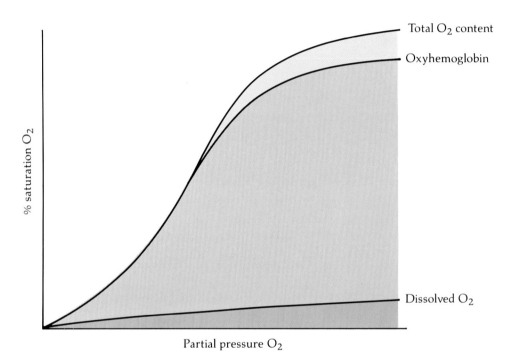

larger amounts of CO_2 are moved chemically as bicarbonate. In addition, CO_2 may be carried in the following ways:

■ As bicarbonate (60% to 70% of the total CO_2)

■ Combined with proteins (20% to 30% of the total CO_2)

■ As dissolved CO_2 (5% to 10% of the total CO_2)

■ A very small amount as carbonic acid (H_2CO_3) (.001% of the total CO_2)

Carbon dioxide is carried in all four of these forms in both the plasma and the red blood cells. However, for CO_2 to form bicarbonate it must first undergo the following chemical reaction:

$$CO_2 + H_2O \longrightarrow H_2CO_3 \longrightarrow (H^+) + (HCO_3^-)$$

This reaction is very slow, occurring in about 20 seconds in the plasma. In the red blood cell, however, the reaction is greatly enhanced by the catalyst carbonic anhydrase and reaction time is reduced to about 0.1 second. As a result, the great majority of bicarbonate is produced first within the red blood cell and then diffuses out of the cell and into the plasma. To maintain electrical and chemical equilibrium as the bicarbonate ion moves out of the cell, this negative ion is exchanged for a chloride ion in the plasma, a transaction referred to as the "chloride shift".

Once CO_2 reaches the lung, the entire reaction involving bicarbonate must occur in reverse in order for the lung to expel CO_2 in a gaseous form. Much larger amounts of CO_2 than O_2 are carried in the blood. The arterial blood contains about 48 vol% CO_2. By contrast, less than half that amount, or 20 vol% O_2, is carried in the arterial blood.

Blood content curves may be constructed for both O_2 and CO_2. Even though it is customary to report CO_2 content in milliequivalents per liter, for comparison purposes both gases are expressed in vol% on the vertical axis. Several important concepts can be illustrated by the curves (Figure 1.25):

■ The content difference between arterial and venous blood for both gases is 5 vol%. In other words, 5 vol% of O_2 is released in the capillary in exchange for 5 vol% of CO_2. The same exchange ratio exists in the lung where 5 vol% of O_2 is added to the venous blood and 5 vol% of CO_2 is released and removed through ventilation. This unique relationship helps to explain how the external gas exchange process must be adjusted to meet the internal gas exchange process for the organism to survive.

■ The change in partial pressure required to add or remove gas is considerably different for each gas. For O_2, the partial pressure climbs from 40 mm Hg in the venous blood to 100 mm Hg in the arterial blood (a difference of 60 mm Hg) to accommodate the addition of 5 vol% O_2. For CO_2, the partial pressure of venous blood must increase by only 6 mm Hg in order to accommodate 5 vol% CO_2 in the tissue.

These pressure differences produce both advantages and disadvantages. The advantage is that large amounts of CO_2 can be readily removed from the lung by simply increasing ventilation by a small amount. Similarly, small increases in the P_{CO_2} of the ve-

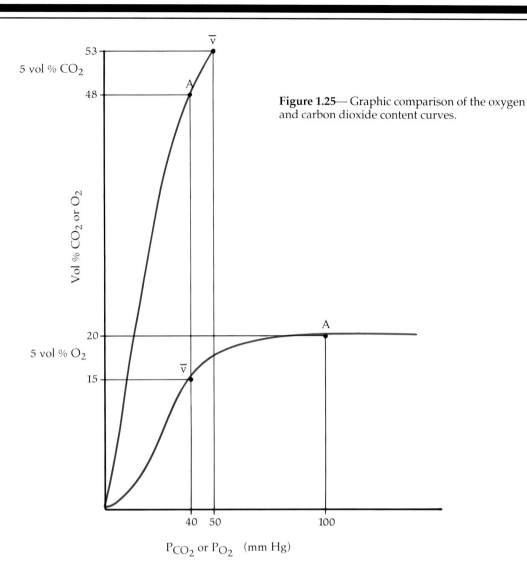

5 vol % CO_2

5 vol % O_2

Vol % CO_2 or O_2

P_{CO_2} or P_{O_2} (mm Hg)

Figure 1.25— Graphic comparison of the oxygen and carbon dioxide content curves.

Figure 1.26— Schematic of the neural activity recorded from the diaphragm illustrating the inspiratory and expiratory components of the breathing cycle.

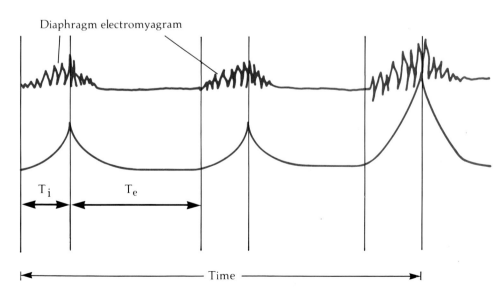

Diaphragm electromyagram

T_i T_e

Time

nous blood can accommodate large amounts of CO_2 production in the tissue capillary which comes into play, for example, during exercise.

Oxygen uptake, on the other hand, is limited in the lung because further increases in partial pressure beyond 100 mm Hg add very little to the O_2 content of the arterial blood. The shape of the O_2 content curve becomes very flat beyond 100 mm Hg, indicating that the hemoglobin molecules are, for the most part, already saturated with O_2 (Figure 1.24). The 100% saturation actually occurs at a PO_2 of 150 mm Hg. However, for practical purposes the curve becomes fairly flat long before this. In terms of O_2 unloading at the tissue, the larger partial pressures confer an advantage because most of the O_2 is unloaded while the partial pressure remains fairly high. High partial pressure facilitates the diffusion of O_2 into the tissue.

1.20 *Control of Ventilation*

Ventilation is controlled by a complex set of systems that involve both voluntary control from the cerebral cortex as well as involuntary, or autonomic, control from the brain stem. Some 25 different sensory mechanisms feed into the brain stem to control ventilation. The primary mechanisms include both chemical and mechanical sensors that provide feedback to the control mechanism. The ventilatory control system, like many of the body's control systems, is regulated primarily through negative feedback mechanisms. The respiratory control center in the medulla of the brainstem sends impulses to the respiratory muscles which produce ventilation. Sensors that respond to the mechanical movement of the lung and chest wall, as well as several chemical sensors that monitor the blood levels of O_2, CO_2, and hydrogen ion, all feed information back to the respiratory control center to modify ventilation. In addition to the sensory systems that modify the respiratory cycle, the respiratory center has some of its own inherent rhythmicity.

1.21 *Ventilatory Cycle*

The ventilatory cycle can be divided into two components, an inspiratory cycle (Ti) and an expiratory cycle (Te). The respiratory control center in the medulla contains nerve fibers that fire predominantly during inspiration (inspiratory neurons) and other fibers that fire only during expiration (expiratory neurons). The tidal volume is a function of both the muscular effort or drive exerted during the breath and the length of the inspiratory cycle. The total cycle and its components (Ti and Te) can be observed by recording the neural impulses from the phrenic nerve, which innervates the diaphragm (Figure 1.26).

1.22 *Chemical and Mechanical Receptors*

Ventilatory control is normally influenced by both chemical (for example, pH, PO_2, PCO_2) and mechanical factors (for example, lung volume, muscle tension in the chest wall and diaphragm).

Two sets of chemoreceptors influence the ventilatory cycle, the central chemoreceptors and the peripheral chemoreceptors. The central chemoreceptors reside on the ventrolateral surface of the medulla and are sensitive only to changes in the pH of the cerebral spinal fluid (CSF) in which they are bathed. Normally, hydrogen ions (H^+) and bicarbonate ions (HCO_3^-) in the blood do not reach these receptors because of the blood brain barrier. However, CO_2 from the blood readily diffuses across the barrier and into the csf, indi-

Figure 1.27— Location of the central and peripheral chemo-receptors.

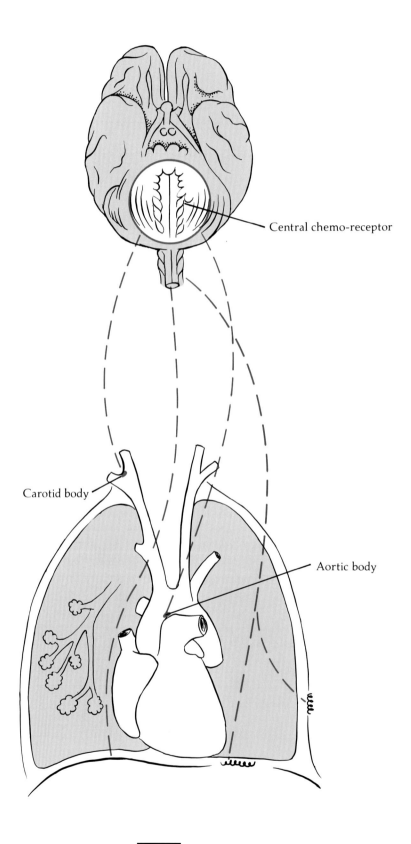

Central chemo-receptor

Carotid body

Aortic body

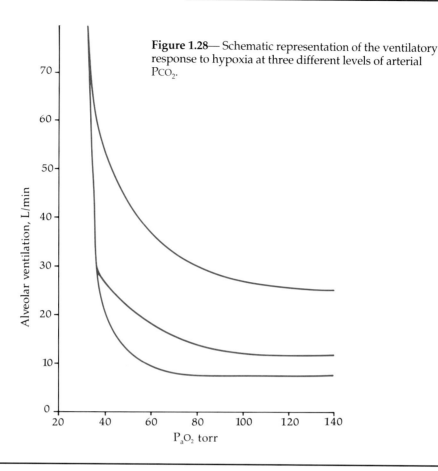

Figure 1.28— Schematic representation of the ventilatory response to hypoxia at three different levels of arterial P_{CO_2}.

rectly stimulating the receptor via the following reaction:

$$CO_2 + H_2O \longrightarrow H_2CO_3 \longrightarrow H^+ + HCO_3^-$$

The hydrogen ion produced in this reaction stimulates the central chemoreceptors, which in turn affect the medullary respiratory center, causing an increase in both tidal volume and breathing frequency. Normally, the cerebral spinal fluid has a pH of about 7.32 which is slightly more acidic than the normal blood pH of 7.40. The cerebral spinal fluid has fewer protein buffers than blood, therefore, small changes in CO_2 diffusing from the blood into the cerebral spinal fluid cause greater changes in pH, which acts as an amplification system. The peripheral chemoreceptors are sensitive to low O_2 tension, high P_aCO_2, and increased hydrogen concentration. Of these variables, low O_2 tension is the most important factor. These receptors are called the carotid and aortic bodies and are located in the arterial system at the bifurcation of the common carotid artery and at the level of the aortic arch (Figure 1.27). Peripheral chemoreceptors influence the respiratory center by changing tidal volume or respiratory drive, rather than by changing respiratory rate. The partial pressure of O_2 in the arterial blood is sensed by the receptors. However, the receptor shows little activity until the O_2 tension has dropped below 60 mm Hg (Figure 1.28). This result correlates with the oxyhemoglobin curve because, below an O_2 tension of 60 mm Hg, the hemoglobin molecule begins to desaturate. It is also the partial pressure below which insurance companies will reimburse for O_2 therapy. Thus, it has both physiologic significance as well as financial implications.

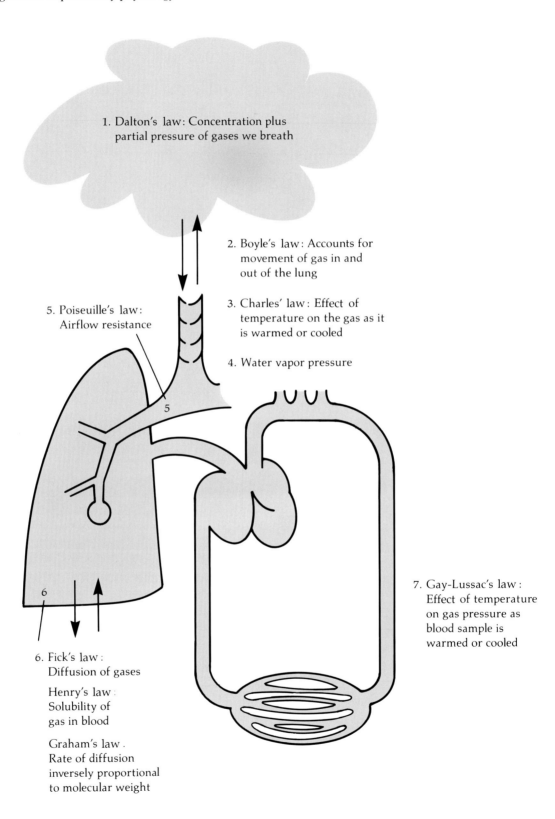

Figure 1.29— Schematic illustrating the impact of the gas laws on pulmonary physiology.

1. Dalton's law: Concentration plus partial pressure of gases we breath

2. Boyle's law: Accounts for movement of gas in and out of the lung

3. Charles' law: Effect of temperature on the gas as it is warmed or cooled

4. Water vapor pressure

5. Poiseuille's law: Airflow resistance

6. Fick's law: Diffusion of gases

Henry's law: Solubility of gas in blood

Graham's law: Rate of diffusion inversely proportional to molecular weight

7. Gay-Lussac's law: Effect of temperature on gas pressure as blood sample is warmed or cooled

The lung has three types of mechanoreceptors that send information back to the respiratory control center to help regulate tidal volume and frequency as well as initiate several important pulmonary reflexes. These include pulmonary stretch receptors, irritant receptors, and juxtacapillary receptors.

Pulmonary stretch receptors are located throughout the lung, in the smooth muscle of the conducting airways, and probably in the periphery of the lung close to the gas exchange region. These receptors are sensitive to stretch as the result of changes in lung volume or pressure. Their firing frequency increases in response to stretch and exhibits a continuous discharge proportional to the amount of volume contained in the FRC. Stimulation of the mechanoreceptor alters the breathing pattern in several different ways:

- During tidal breathing as lung volume increases, stimulation of the receptor (once the stimulus is transmitted to the respiratory control center) causes reflex inhibition that terminates the tidal breath.

- The continuous discharge at static lung volumes (FRC) helps to delay the onset of the next inspiration, thus prolonging the expiratory phase. This reflex is called the Hering-Breuer reflex, described as prolongation of the respiratory cycle produced by maintaining lung inflation.

- The pulmonary stretch receptors are also responsible for the deflation reflex — a decrease in lung volume causing a decrease in stretch receptor activity, thus removing the inhibitory action of the pulmonary stretch receptors and causing the next inspiration to occur. Deflation of the lung also stimulates inspiratory efforts.

Irritant receptors are primarily located in the upper airways and in the region of the carina. These receptors respond to changes in lung volume (ΔV) during inspiration and expiration. They do not respond to static lung volumes. They are called irritant receptors because they respond to inhaled particles (for example, dust and smoke) and to chemical irritants (for example, ammonia and sulfur dioxide), resulting in the initiation of the cough reflex. Stimulation of the irritant receptor also causes an increase in ventilation by affecting the drive component and probably also affects the breathing rate. Finally, the irritant receptors initiate bronchoconstriction, a mechanism that would presumably narrow airways to increase the velocity of air expulsion during cough. They may, however, have a negative role in the cause of exercise-induced asthma.

Juxtacapillary receptors (J receptors) are located close to the pulmonary capillary. They respond to certain types of drug ingestion, but their main stimulus is capillary congestion as seen in pulmonary edema. Sensitization of receptor causes several responses which may be interpreted as physiologic adjustments to compensate for pulmonary congestion: stimulation of ventilation, inhibition of somatic or muscle activity, systemic vasodilation, and bradycardia.

1.23 *Physics of Gases*

The physiology of lung function involves numerous applications of the fundamental properties of gases and the physical laws that determine their behavior. These laws apply to the gases we breathe (warming, cooling, humidity, partial pressures), to the process of ventilation (compression and decompression of the gases), to the distribution of the gases through the lung (pressures required to produce flow), to the resistances encountered during flow, and to the diffusion of gases across the lung membrane and into the blood. Figure 1.29 presents a brief summary of the applications related to pulmonary physiology.

1.24   *Kinetic Theory of Gases*

Four statements comprise the kinetic theory of gases:

- A gas that occupies a space is not continuous, but rather consists of an enormous number of discrete particles or molecules that have mass. According to Avogadro's law (see below) any gas at standard temperature and pressure contains 6.023×10^{23} molecules and occupies 22.4 liters or 6.023×10^{23} / 22.4 liters = 26×10^{18}/cc = 26,000,000,000,000,000,000 molecules/cc.

- Gas molecules are in constant motion. Because they move and have mass, they have kinetic energy ($E = 1/2\ Mv^2$).

- Gas molecules continually collide with one another. They rebound from these collisions without loss of energy, and are, therefore, called elastic collisions. Gas molecules do not attract each other: i.e., there are no van der Waals forces or cohesive forces between gas molecules.

- Gas particles have kinetic energy that, when added together, form pressure. At a given temperature, the product $1/2\ Mv^2 = E$ is the same for all gases.

    For gases that have the same concentration or same number of particles in a container, the pressure will be identical regardless of the type of gas if the temperature remains the same. This also means that, for a given temperature, the particles of a lighter gas must travel faster in order for the kinetic energy to be the same.

1.25   *Avogadro's Law*

Equal volumes of gases at the same temperature and pressure contain the same number of molecules. Or, conversely, at constant temperature and pressure equal numbers of molecules of all gases occupy the same volume.

    The weights of all molecules corresponding to their molecular weights or gram atomic weights contain the same number of particles: 6.023×10^{23}. This is known as Avogadro's number.

    At standard temperature and pressure, one gram molecular weight of a gas contains 6.023×10^{26} molecules and occupies 22.4 liters.

1.26   *General Gas Law*

The general gas law (sometimes also referred to as the ideal gas law) states the relationship between temperature pressure and volume for a gas.

$$PV = nRT \qquad \text{Equation 1.11}$$

where

n = mass or number of gas molecules
R = gas constant that varies depending on the units of measure selected.
T = absolute temperature
P = pressure
V = volume.

In pulmonary physiology, the applications of the general gas law do not involve changing the gas constant nor the mass of the gas under consideration.

As a result, the above equation can be expressed as:

$$\frac{PV}{T} = nR \qquad \text{Equation 1.12}$$

where (nR) is now considered a constant.

$$\frac{P_1 V_1}{T_1} = nR = \frac{P_2 V_2}{T_2} \qquad \text{Equation 1.13}$$

Equation 1.13 is frequently used as a working equation to determine how a gas sample under a set of initial conditions for temperature pressure and volume will change when exposed to a new set of conditions. In actuality, the initial relationships were derived by holding one of the three variables constant and determining the relationship between the other two.

The following three gas laws may be derived simply by selecting one of the variables as a constant.

1.26.1 Boyle's Law

When **temperature** is held constant, the volume of a gas varies inversely with the pressure.

For temperature constant:
$$P_1 V_1 = (nRT) \text{ "constant"} \qquad \text{Equation 1.14}$$

where
$$P_1 V_1 = (nRT) = P_2 V_2$$

$$V_2 = \frac{V_1 P_1}{P_2}$$

This relationship accounts for the movement of gases in and out of the lung. During inspiration, expansion of the thorax causes the pressure inside the lung to decrease, resulting in movement of gas into the lung. During expiration, compression of the gas in the lung causes the pressure to increase above atmospheric and gas then flows out of the lung.

An interesting result of Boyle's law is the effect that underwater depths have on the lung volumes. Table 1.1 illustrates the lung volumes that would result from diving to certain depths while holding one's breath. The critical observation for scuba divers is that the lung volume doubles in ascending from 33 feet to the surface. It is, therefore, essential that the diver continue to exhale slowly while ascending.

Table 1.1—Lung volumes at certain depths of water.

Surface	P_2	V_2	P_1V_1 = Constant	$V_2 = \dfrac{P_1V_1}{P_2}$
0 ft.	1 ATM	12 qts.	1 x 12 = 12	$V_2 = 1/1\,(12)$
33 ft.	2 ATM	6 qts.	2 x 6 = 12	$V_2 = 1/2\,(12)$
66 ft.	3 ATM	4 qts.	3 x 4 = 12	$V_2 = 1/3\,(12)$
99 ft.	4 ATM	3 qts.	4 x 3 = 12	$V_2 = 1/4\,(12)$
132 ft.	5 ATM	2.4 qts.	5 x 2.4 = 12	$V_2 = 1/5\,(12)$

1.26.2 Charles' Law

When **pressure** is held constant, the volume of a gas is directly proportional to the temperature.

For pressure constant:
$$PV_1 = nRT_1 \text{ or } \frac{V_1}{T_1} = \frac{nR}{P} \text{ "constant"} \qquad \textbf{Equation 1.15}$$

$$\frac{V_1}{T_1} = \frac{nR}{P} = \frac{V_2}{T_2}$$

$$V_2 = \frac{V_1 T_2}{T_1}$$

Charles' law is frequently used during pulmonary function testing where lung volumes are measured at room temperature and then converted to the lung volume that exists at body temperature. For example, when breathing air in the arctic, if the outside temperature is 50° F below zero (temperatures encountered during the Iditerod trail run), the air warmed to body temperature would undergo approximately a 50% increase in volume.

1.26.3 Gay-Lussac's Law

When **volume** is held constant, the pressure exerted by a gas varies directly with the absolute temperature.

Volume Constant:
$$VP_1 = nRT_1 \text{ or } \frac{P_1}{T_1} = \frac{nR}{V} \text{ "constant"} \qquad \textbf{Equation 1.16}$$

$$\frac{P_1}{T_1} = \frac{nR}{V} = \frac{P_2}{T_2}$$

$$P_2 = \frac{P_1 T_2}{T_1}$$

This law has applications during the measurement of blood gases in the laboratory setting. Blood samples are customarily transported on ice at approximately 0 degrees centigrade. The blood sample is injected into a machine that warms the blood to body temperature and measures the partial pressures of the gases (O_2 and CO_2) in the blood. As the sample gradually warms, the pressures exerted by the gases in the sample also increase.

1.27 *Dalton's Law of Partial Pressures*

The total pressure exerted by a mixture of gases equals the sum of the partial pressure of the constituent gases. The partial pressure of each gas in the mixture is the pressure each gas would exert if it alone occupied the volume.

$$V_P = V(P_1 + P_2 + P_3 + ... + P_n) \qquad \textbf{Equation 1.17}$$

$$P_{Total} = (P_1 + P_2 + P_3 + ... + P_n)$$

Therefore, each gas in a mixture contributes its share of the total pressure of the mixture in proportion to its percentage or concentration in the mixture.

Dalton's law of partial pressures has tremendous clinical applications because the pressures exerted by certain gases can be altered by changing the concentration of the gas. Specifically, patients often receive higher concentrations of O_2 to breath because this increases the partial pressure of O_2 in the lung. This, in turn, facilitates the movement of O_2 into the pulmonary blood and increases the total amount of O_2 carried to the tissue.

Water Vapor: Water exists primarily as a liquid at room temperature. However, water molecules are constantly escaping from the surface of the water to form water vapor. As these molecules escape, they also begin to exert a partial pressure. The rate at which the molecules escape is a function of temperature. Water continues to evaporate until the rate of leaving equals the rate of return. This equilibrium point is a function of the temperature alone. Therefore, temperature determines the partial pressure of water in a gaseous mixture.

1.28 *Diffusion*

Several laws influence the rate at which gases move from the alveolar gas space and into the blood space, including Henry's law, Graham's law, and Fick's law.

1.28.1 Henry's Law

The quantity of gas that dissolves in a liquid is proportional to partial pressure and solubility:

- The quantity of gas that dissolves increases in a linear fashion with partial pressure (provided that the gas does not react with the solvent).

■ The quantity of gas dissolved is related to partial pressure by the solubility coefficient (solubility is inversely related to temperature).

Solubility of gases in liquids is generally reported in volumes percent or the amount of a gas in milliliters that is dissolved in 100 milliliters of solvent.

$$\text{Vol\%} = \frac{\text{volume of a gas in mls}}{100 \text{ mls of solvent}}$$

The solubility coefficient of O_2 in whole blood is calculated from the Busen solubility coefficient:

Solubility of O_2 in blood = .023 mls of O_2 dissolves in each ml of plasma for every 760 mm Hg pressure.

Converting to the more generally accepted units of vol%:

Solubility of O_2 in blood = .003 mls of O_2/100 mls blood /1 mm Hg

The amount of O_2 that dissolves in blood at any partial pressure is then:

$$\text{Vol\%} = P_{O_2} \times .003$$

The solubility of coefficient of CO_2 in whole blood can be similarly reported:

Solubility of CO_2 in blood = 0.47 mls of CO_2 dissolves in each ml of blood for every 760 mm Hg.

Converting to units of vol%:

Solubility of CO_2 in blood = 0.67 vol% for each mm Hg
(as can be seen by comparison of their respective solubilities, CO_2 is much more soluble in blood than O_2).

In the laboratory, dissolved CO_2 is often reported as millimoles (mM)/liter of plasma, or

Solubility of CO_2 in mM/l = $P_{CO_2} \times 0.03$

The mM/liter can be converted to vol% by multiplying by 2.23, (or mM/liter = vol% / 2.23).

See Table 1.2 for the solubilities of other gases in blood or plasma.

Table 1.2—Solubility Coefficients of Gases at 38° C

Gas	SOLVENT			
	Water	Plasma	Red Cell	Blood*
H_2	0.0162	0.0153	0.0145	0.0149
He	0.00085	–	–	0.0087
N_2	0.0127	0.0117	0.0146	0.0130
O_2	0.0232	0.0209	0.0261	0.0230
CO	0.01816	–	–	–
CO_2	0.545	0.510	0.44	0.47

*Assuming a hematocrit of 45% with O_2 capacity of 20 vol%

1.28.2 Graham's Law

The relative rates of diffusion of gases (under the same conditions) are inversely proportional to the square roots of the molecular weights (MW).

$$\dot{V} \text{ is proportional to } \frac{1}{\text{square root of MW}}$$

Graham's law may be considered as an application of the kinetic theory of gases: for diffusion of gases within a gaseous medium at a given temperature, smaller particles move faster and collide more frequently and diffuse faster.

Table 1.3 presents a comparison of relative rates of diffusion based on Graham's law.

Table 1.3—The rate of a gas varies inversely as the square roots of their molecular weights at similar temperatures and pressures.

Gas	Molecular Weight
Hydrogen	2.01
Helium	4.00
Nitrogen	28.01
Ethylene	28.04
Oxygen	32.00
Carbon Dioxide	44.01
Nitrous Oxide	44.01

1.28.3 Fick's Law

Fick's law combines a number of factors, including the properties of both Henry's law and Graham's law, to describe the transfer of gases across biologic membranes such as tissue capillaries and the alveolar capillary membrane (Figure 1.30).

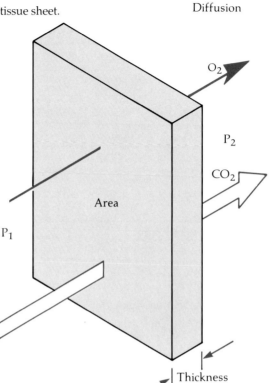

Figure 1.30— Diffusion through a tissue sheet.

Diffusion

O_2

P_2

CO_2

Area

P_1

Thickness

Fick's law:

$$\text{Rate of transfer of a gas } (\dot{V}gas) = \frac{A\,D\,(P_1 - P_2)}{t}$$ **Equation 1.18**

where

A = cross-sectional area of the membrane across which the diffusion occurs.

D = diffusion coefficient is proportional to the solubility and inversely proportional to the square root of the molecular weight.

$(P_1 - P_2)$ = pressure gradient across the membrane

t = thickness of the membrane.

1.29   *Poiseuille's Law*

Poiseuille's law describes the relation between pressure, flow, and resistance for fluids and gases. It is the fluidic analogue of Ohm's law.

$$E = I \times R \quad \text{or} \quad I = E/R$$

$$P = \dot{V} \times R \quad \text{or} \quad \text{Flow} = P/R$$

Poiseuille's law: $$\text{Flow} = \frac{(P_1 - P_2)\,\pi\,r^4}{8\,l\,n}$$ **Equation 1.19** where $(P_1 - P_2)$ = the pressure gradient across the tube

$$\frac{1}{R} = \frac{\pi r^4}{8 l n}$$

or $$R = \frac{8 l n}{\pi r^4}$$

Poiseuille's law only applies to conditions of laminar flow. For the conditions of turbulent flow, the pressure required to produce the same amount of flow increases in proportion to a constant times the flow of the gas squared. For gas flow in the lung, which is a combination of both laminar and turbulent conditions, the pressure required to produce flow can be expressed as (Figure 1.31):

$$P = K_1 \dot{V} + K_2 \dot{V}^2 \qquad \qquad \textbf{Equation 1.20}$$

where K = constant
$\dot{V}$ = flow.

Poiseuille's law has a number of applications in pulmonary physiology:

■ Measurement of airflow resistance has applications to the clinical setting with patients on mechanical ventilators (Section 1.11). In addition, airflow resistance can be measured noninvasively in the body with a plethysmograph by determining the pressure difference between the mouth pressure and the alveolar pressure.

■ Many flow transducers which are a part of a number of medical monitoring devices apply Poiseuille's law. They measure flow by determining the pressure difference across a fixed resistance. The airway response to drug therapy (bronchodilator drugs) can be roughly measured using a peak flow meter. This device works in a similar fashion to the flow transducer. A fixed resistor is placed in the tube and moves according to the pressure difference created by the flow. The pressure difference across the tube moves the resistor in proportion to the flow through the tube.

■ Air flow is distributed in the lung according to several mechanisms that control airway caliber including neural control (sympathetic and parasympathetic innervation), reflexes, humoral substances, and dilation in response to airway CO_2. These mechanisms control local ventilation very much in the same fashion as smooth muscle bands control capillary circulation through the precapillary sphincters.

■ Obstructive lung disorders are characterized by changes in the flow properties of the airways. Frequently, these changes result from alterations in the dimensions or resistance characteristic of the airway.

Figure 1.31— Resistance to air flow through tubes.

Laminar

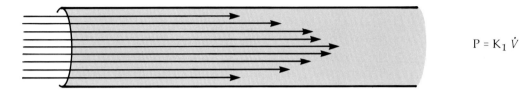

$P = K_1 \dot{V}$

Turbulent

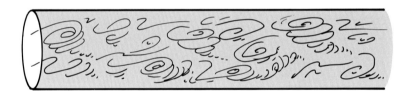

$P = K_2 \dot{V}^2$

Tracheo-bronchial

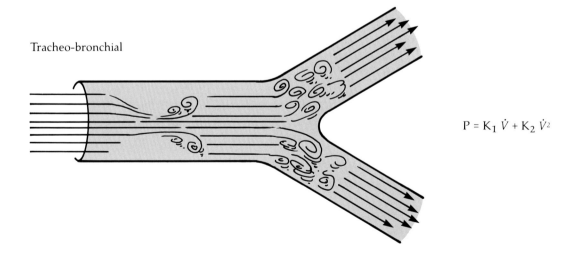

$P = K_1 \dot{V} + K_2 \dot{V}^2$

2.0 AIRWAY MONITORING OF ADULT, PEDIATRIC, AND NEONATAL PATIENTS

Many health care workers including respiratory care practitioners, cardiopulmonary technologists and technicians, physicians, and nurses work with respiratory mechanical concepts every day. Parameters such as volume, flow, and pressure are used to quantitatively classify the mechanical status of the patient's airways and lungs. This section presents and discusses the information obtained from noninvasive monitoring of the airway of adult, pediatric, or neonatal patients. Each subsection describes the devices used to measure the basic physiologic parameters and describes their principles of operation as well as some clinical considerations.

Separate issues such as standards of performance, calibration requirements, infection control procedures, and specifications for adult, pediatric, and neonatal devices are beyond the scope of this section. The American Association for Respiratory Care and the American Thoracic Society have published recommendations and guidelines and developed measurement standards for respiratory and pulmonary function devices. Managers of Respiratory Therapy and Pulmonary Laboratories are familiar with these standards and practices and can refer the reader to appropriate documentation for further information.

2.1 *Volume Monitoring*

Respiratory volumes are usually measured and expressed in liters. One liter equals 1.06 quarts. Smaller volumes are expressed in milliliters. One liter contains 1,000 milliliters. Prior to the introduction of the third generation of mechanical ventilators, the graphic representation of volume was not available as an analog output, but as a mechanical output as exemplified by the following devices (which are still in use today). Modern pulmonary function systems and ventilators now present volume measurement related to flow, pressure, and time. Flow-volume, pressure-volume, and volume-time relationships (loops) help related pathophysiology to normal standards for diagnosis and differentiation of pulmonary diseases and disorders. Refer to the Section 8.0 for references.

2.1.1 Mechanical Air-Turbine Meter

A rotating vane spirometer, such as the Wright Respirometer™, uses a flat two-bladed rotor, or vane, running in jeweled bearings. As gas enters the turbine meter, a series of slots directs the air flow to the vane. The vane is connected to the hands of a dial through a watch-type movement containing a series of gears. The vane rotates unidirectionally as the volume registers on the face of a dial calibrated in liters (Figure 2.1).

Clinical considerations: Generally used as a portable unit, the mechanical air turbine meter has some inherent limitations. It has a resistance to flow of 2 cm of water (H_2O) because 2 to 3 liters per minute (LPM) of airflow are required to turn the vanes. The resistance to flow before the vanes begin to turn can be considered as a measure of sensitivity. A turbine meter of high sensitivity would have a low resistance to flow. Similarly, a device of low sensitivity would have a high resistance to flow. Because of the nonlinear response to flow, this measurement is affected considerably by the waveform of the gas flowing through it. Therefore, a short, sharp breath will give a higher reading than a long, slow

Figure 2.1— The mechanical air turbine meter.

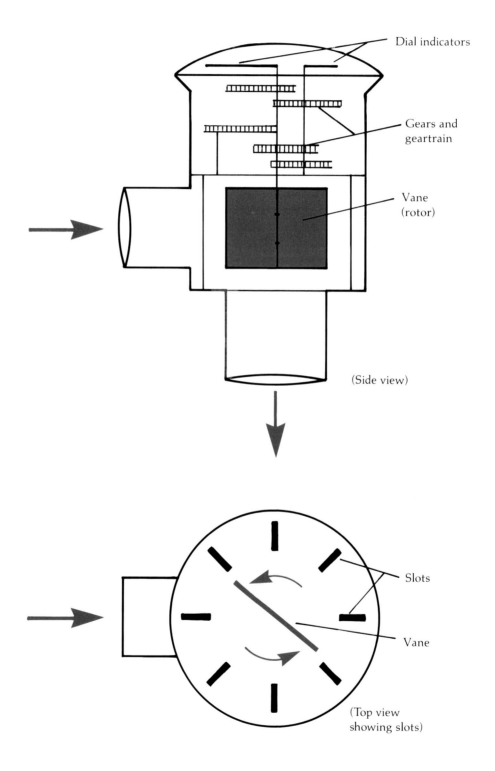

Dial indicators

Gears and geartrain

Vane (rotor)

(Side view)

Slots

Vane

(Top view showing slots)

Figure 2.2— The electronic air turbine meter.

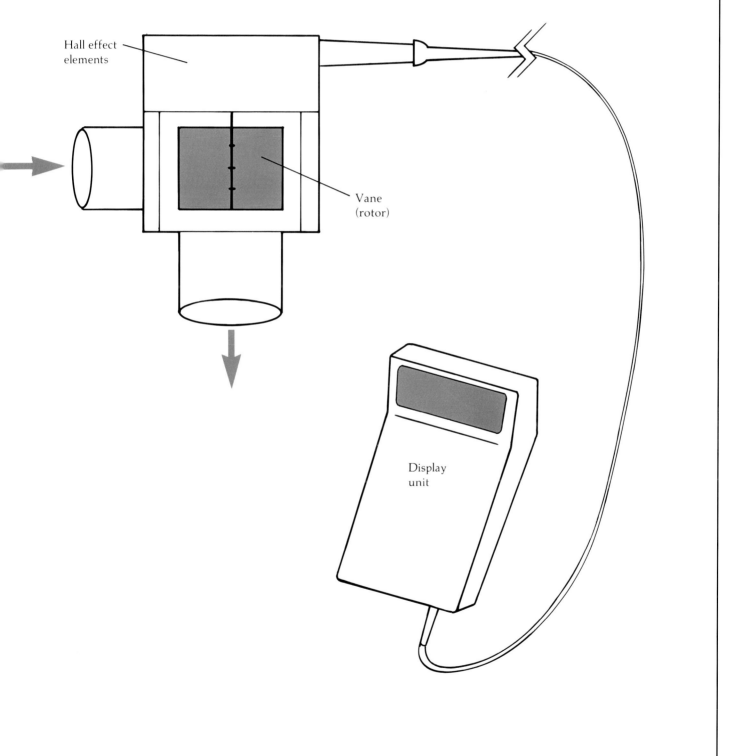

Figure 2.3— Ultrasonic vortex sensor.

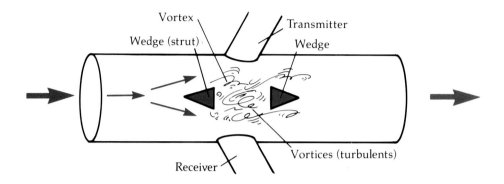

Figure 2.4— Hot wire anemometer.

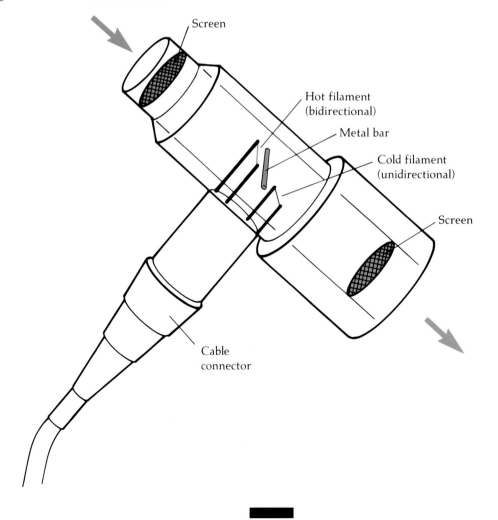

breath of equal volume. The mechanical air turbine meter also has a deadspace of 22 milliliters and a maximum flow of 300 LPM. Flows in excess of 300 LPM, as observed while performing a forced expiratory volume (FEV) maneuver, will permanently damage the vanes. Due to the large deadspace and low sensitivity, this device is unsuitable for neonates and small children. The turbine meter remains adequate for routine volume screening in adults, as long as its limitations are understood.

2.1.2   Electronic Air-Turbine Meter

This device, represented by the Wright Magtrak™, is the electronic version of the turbine meter. The upper gear train and dials have been replaced with an encapsulated circuit board and Hall Effect element. Magnetism is used as a transducer and electronic pulses are transmitted as the vane rotates. The pulses are interpreted and relayed to the hand-held unit that displays tidal volume, minute volume, and breaths per minute (Figure 2.2).

     Clinical considerations: The accuracy, sensitivity, resistance to flow, and deadspace are identical to the mechanical air turbine meter. Turbines using titanium vanes for the maximum flow can be extended to 700 LPM. Because the hand-held display unit contains microprocessors, information is easier to obtain than with the mechanical meter.

2.2   *Flow Monitoring*

Flow is generally defined as a volume transferred per unit of time. It is expressed as liters per second (l/sec). As with small volumes, small flows can be expressed in milliliters per second (ml/sec) or milliliters per minute (ml/min). Flow measurement, as well as pressure and volume measurement, usually occurs in the circuit of the ventilator in the inspiratory limb, in the expiratory limb, or in both limbs.

2.2.1   Ultrasonic Sensing of Vortices

One of the more interesting flow detection methods involves the creation of vortices. A vortex forms when a partial obstruction, such as a wedge or strut, is placed in the stream of gas flowing through a tube. The resulting turbulents vibrate from side to side along the length of the tube. The greater the velocity of the air stream, the faster the vibrations in the tube. The wedge is designed to generate one beat (vortex) for each milliliter of gas that passes through the tube (Figure 2.3).

     The vortices, or turbulents, are sensed by an ultrasonic beam placed perpendicular to the direction of gas flow. An electronically-powered crystal transducer sends the ultrasonic beam across the tube to a receiver. The created vortices intermittently change the strength of the ultrasonic beam. The receiver converts the changes, or counts, into an electronic signal directly proportional to flow. Tidal volume and minute volume can be calculated from the flow rate.

     Clinical considerations: The location and number of vortices is unaffected by the composition, density, temperature, or humidity of the gas. With continued use in high humidity environments, the flow transducer has a tendency to accumulate condensed water on the transmitter and receiver domes. This water acts as an obstruction to the transmitter/receiver signal and can cause erratic or incorrect volume readings.

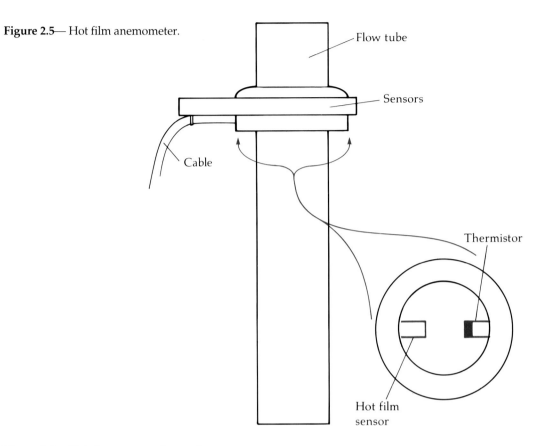

Figure 2.5— Hot film anemometer.

Figure 2.6— Fleisch pneumotachograph.

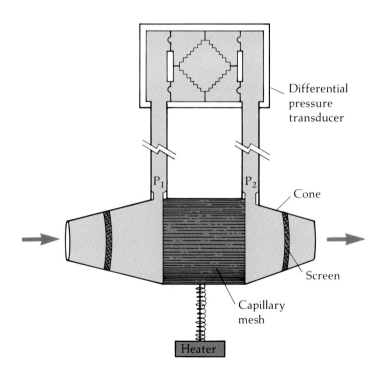

The major disadvantage of this type of flow sensor is that it has a minimum flow sensing threshold of 5 LPM which makes it unsuitable for neonatal measurements. In addition, it senses flow bidirectionally and, therefore, does not work in some environments unless a one-way valve is placed in-line.

Examples of equipment that use the ultrasonic vortex principle are the Bourns LS-75® and its successor the VM-90, the Bourns LS-80®, and the Bear® I, II, III, and V ventilators.

2.2.2   Hot-Wire Anemometer

Anemometry (from Greek, "wind measure") first described by Utenick and used by Godal, is based on the fact that a heated filament exposed to a flow of gas will lose heat.[1,2] The rate of heat loss varies with the velocity of the gas. The anemometer, as exemplified by the sensor of the Bear Neonatal Volume Monitor (NVM-1)®, has two filaments, one cold and one hot.[3] The filaments are usually platinum because this metal does not react with many chemicals. The cold filament measures the gas temperature and regulates a current through the hot filament. That current regulates the heating of the hot filament so that a constant temperature difference is maintained between the two filaments by the current (Figure 2.4).

As the gas flow enters the tube, the hot filament, typically at 50 degrees centigrade, cools. The heating current increases to maintain the temperature difference. The increase in the current is proportional to the flow of the gas through the tube. The signal can be integrated to calculate the inspired tidal volume, expired tidal volume, and % tube leakage.

Clinical considerations: Anemometry has some advantages over pneumotachography in that it is not significantly affected by low or high flow rates. Very high flow rates, however, will create turbulents that disturb the results. The major advantage of this particular device is that it can be used with neonates. It has a deadspace of only four cubic centimeters and a flow range of between 0.15 to 21 LPM. The major disadvantage of anemometry is that, since it lies in the mainstream of the airway and is usually placed as close to the patient "Y" as possible, it may become partially obstructed with mucus. When mucus adheres to the wire filament, false flow readings may occur. As with the ultrasonic-vortex type of flow sensor, the hot wire anemometer can be inaccurate in high humidity environments. An adult ventilator called the Bear 1000, currently under development, uses the adult version of the hot wire anemometer to determine expiratory flow rate.

2.2.3   Hot-Film Anemometer

An example of the hot film anemometer is the flow sensor of the Puritan Bennett 7200® series microprocessor ventilators. Although similar flow transducers measure flow through the O_2 and air solenoids, the exhalation flow transducer is of particular interest in this unit. All hot film flow transducers measure the cooling effect of the gas on a heated (200 degrees centigrade) platinum-coated quartz rod that constitutes one side of a resistance bridge circuit. As gas flows across the hot film and cools it, the bridge circuit maintains a constant electrical current by varying the voltage. The voltage is proportional to the flow rate of the gas passing through the transducer. These flow transducers respond over a flow range of 0 to 160 LPM (Figure 2.5).

Because the gas flowing through the flow transducers can differ in temperature, thermistors are mounted on each transducer. Thermistor voltage changes are proportional to the flow rate of the gas passing through the transducer.

Clinical considerations: The hot film anemometer is not as susceptible to flow inaccuracies caused by the expansion and contraction of a metal wire. The addition of temperature compensation to the flow calculations results in a very accurate flow monitoring device. Since the expiratory flow sensor is incorporated in the ventilator located a significant distance from the patient connection, some degradation of the actual flow waveform can occur.

2.3   *Pressure Monitoring*

Pressure is usually defined as a force per unit of area. Force is expressed in the same units as weight, such as pound (lb). Area may be expressed in units such as square feet (ft^2) or square inches (in^2). Therefore, pressure may be expressed as pounds per square inch (lbs/in^2) or, more commonly, PSI. Pressure may also be expressed as millimeters of mercury (mm Hg) or centimeters of water (cm H_2O). These units of length refer to the height to which a column of Hg or H_2O would rise in a close-ended tube under vacuum. Mercury rises under standard atmospheric conditions, temperature, and gravity to a height of 760 millimeters (torr). Mercury is 13.6 times as heavy as an equal volume of H_2O, so under the same conditions, H_2O would rise to a height of 13.6 x 760 mm, or 10,336 mm of H_2O or 33.9 feet. Occasionally, conversions are necessary. A good conversion to remember is: 1 mm Hg = 1.36 cm H_2O.[4]

By measuring the pressure difference across a known resistance during gas movement, flow rates can be calculated and displayed. The Pitot tube, an older device, consists of a tube with a short right-angled bend that orients vertically in the stream of a gas such that the mouth of the bent tube is directed upstream. The Pitot tube is used with a manometer to measure the velocity of the fluid or gas. The more modern pneumotachometers, with screen or heated meshes, are sensitive to gas density and internal pressures.[5] Therefore, they are most accurate with a constant gas composition and internal reference pressure (usually atmospheric) against which they have been calibrated. When used under changing internal pressures and gas compositions, as encountered when using mechanical ventilators, their absolute accuracy may be only ±10%. The signal produced by these units is proportional to flow and can be electronically manipulated (integrated) to provide another signal that is proportional to volume. Remember that a transducer, by definition, is a device that is activated by power from one system and supplies power in another form to a second system. An example would be flow "transducing" a pressure.

2.3.1   Fleisch Pneumotachograph

The Fleisch pneumotachograph consists of a tube with a fixed obstruction, a capillary mesh that produces a slight pressure drop as a flow of gas passes through the device. The pressure created before the mesh (P_1) and after the mesh (P_2) is transmitted to a differential pressure transducer, giving rise to an analog electrical signal proportional to the difference in pressure between P_1 and P_2. The purpose of the cone shape, the screen, and the mesh is to generate a flow pattern that is as laminar as possible since a turbulent flow creates an artificially high pressure differential.[6] The heater heats the mesh so that H_2O vapor does not condense on it (Figure 2.6).

Clinical considerations: The Fleisch pneumotachograph is used to continuously monitor volume, flow, and breathing rates of patients on mechanical ventilators. Since it is sensitive to obstructions, it should not be placed in contact with moisture or secretions from the patient. Its relatively large size and weight can become another drawback during patient monitoring.

2.3.2 Variable Orifice, Flexible Obstruction Transducer

This class of transducers is characterized by an obstruction to flow that deforms, bends, or flexes in response to the gas flow through the device. The various configurations of the flexible obstruction attempt to manufacture a device that produces as linear a flow as possible throughout the full flow range of the transducer.

2.3.3 VarFlex Flow Transducer

The VarFlex™ flow transducer, as incorporated in the CP-100 Pulmonary Monitor manufactured by Bicore Monitoring Systems, is a precision light-weight, bidirectional device that fits within the ventilator circuit. At the core of the device is a wafer-thin austenitic stainless steel "window" with exceptional bending fatigue strength. Due to the unique design of this window, the VarFlex flow transducer is not affected by moisture or respiratory secretions and requires no maintenance, adjustment, or calibration (Figure 2.7).

As gas flows through the transducer, the variable area obstruction window, created by three leaves, deflects in proportion to the gas flow. Because of the shape and location of the leaves, the difference in pressure across the obstruction changes almost linearly with the change in the gas flow rate. The leaves are configured so that they will not interfere with the gas flow.

Clinical considerations: According to the manufacturer, the flow transducer is designed so that the inner walls and leaves are insulated from the ambient temperature. Therefore, condensation does not occur and will not interfere with the accuracy of this unit. The deadspace of 8.6 milliliters in the adult and pediatric units is not acceptable for use in infant and neonatal populations. Infant sensors are presently under development.

2.3.4 Accutach Flow Transducer

The Accutach™ flow transducer, formerly used with the now obsolete Critikon respiratory monitor, is currently used in the Hamilton adult ventilator. This transducer, manufactured by Carlsbad International, is another precision bidirectional, reusable device designed to be placed between the patient connection and the "Y" of the ventilator circuit. The transducer housing contains a thin mylar membrane with a specific design to function as a variable obstruction. The low adherence and high resilience properties of mylar make it optimal for this usage (Figure 2.8).

Clinical considerations: The internal deadspace of the flow transducer is 9 milliliters. This small amount of rebreathed volume will not adversely affect most adult and pediatric patients, but is not acceptable for infants or neonates. Another important aspect of the Accutach flow transducer is that the sensor must be placed so that the pressure sensing tubes are in the vertical (upright) position. If they are in the dependent position, moisture tends to accumulate in them, thus decreasing the accuracy of the device.

Figure 2.7— VarFlex flow transducer.

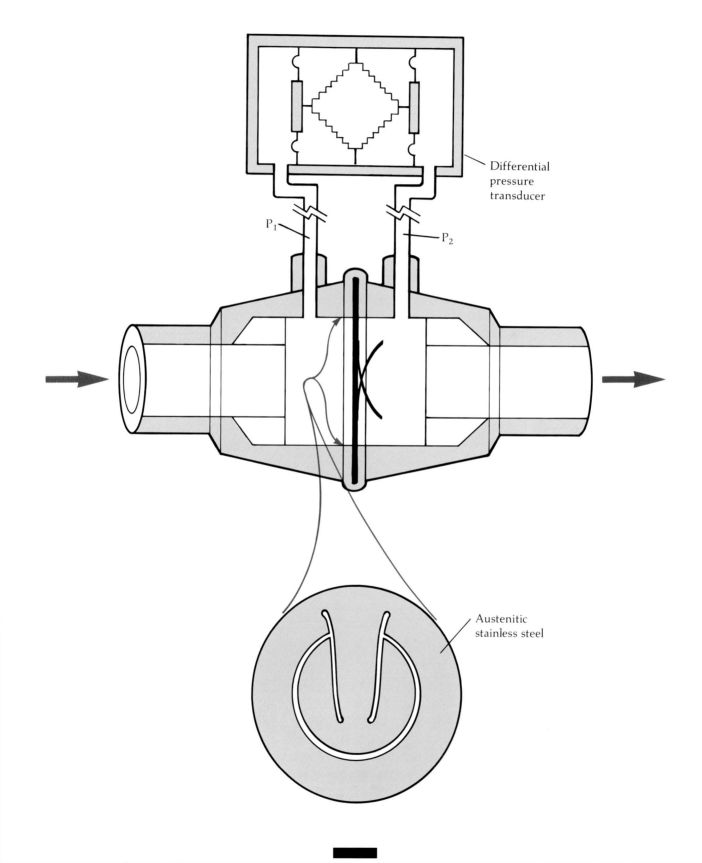

Differential pressure transducer

P_1

P_2

Austenitic stainless steel

2.3.5   Bird Flow Transducer

The Bird® flow transducer is similar in construction to the VarFlex and Accutach devices, except that the variable area obstruction membrane is a nonporous, nonadhesive space age material called Sandvic™. According to the manufacturer, the material has a high tensile strength and an ability to survive multiple flexes for a repeatable resistance to flow and a long life. The window cut into the membrane resembles a flap, but functions like a variable obstruction in the face of variable flows. Wire "cross hairs" are designed to prevent the insertion of cleaning tools that could permanently damage the membrane (Figure 2.9).

      Clinical considerations: The Bird flow transducer is currently incorporated into the Bird® 6400 and 8400 adult ventilators, the VIP infant ventilator, and the Partner™ volume monitor. The Bird Company has released an adult and a pediatric version of the flow transducer — both using the same differential pressure transducer. The flow range for the adult transducer is 4 - 250 LPM; and 2 - 120 LPM for the pediatric transducer. The infant sensor, currently under development, will have a flow range of 0.2 - 20 LPM. The microprocessor is able to distinguish the different types of flow transducers as well as their calibration characteristics by optically reading the holes punched in the connector.

2.4   *Oxygen Analysis/Monitoring*

It is extremely important to determine the O_2 concentration being delivered by the various mechanical devices used to support a patient in respiratory difficulty. Most of the O_2 analyzer/monitors are placed on the inspiratory limb of the ventilator circuit and before the humidifier, if possible, so that the effect of humidity is minimized. The following discussion addresses the more commonly used O_2 analyzer/monitors. As a side note, the difference between an O_2 analyzer and an O_2 monitor is the monitor has the high and low alarm limits built into the unit, whereas the analyzer has no alarms.

2.4.1   Static Paramagnetic Analyzer

Oxygen is unique among gases because it is paramagnetic, which means it is attracted by a magnetic field. Most other gases are diamagnetic, meaning they are repelled or unaffected by a magnetic field. Once in the presence of the magnetic field, O_2 molecules become like small magnets and intensify the strength of the magnetic field, a phenomenon known as Pauling's principle. As exemplified by the Beckman D-2, the paramagnetic analyzer internally contains two small nitrogen-filled spheres assembled to resemble a dumbbell suspended on a taunt, durable quartz fiber between the poles of two nonuniform permanent magnets. The intensity of the two magnetic fields is different so that there is already some torque on the quartz fiber (Figure 2.10).

      Through intermittent sampling, which is technically an invasive procedure, the aspirated gas is dried by passing through silica gel before reaching the measuring area. Oxygen entering the analysis cell increases the torque and, therefore, the rotation of the dumbbell. Attached to the quartz fiber and dumbbell element is a mirror. A light beam, projected onto the mirror, is reflected to a translucent graded scale.

      Clinical considerations: The invasive, intermittent sampling technique results in a prolonged response time. Due to the fragile components used in its construction and because changes in barometric pressure, humidity, extreme temperatures, and variable gas

Figure 2.8— Accutach flow transducer.

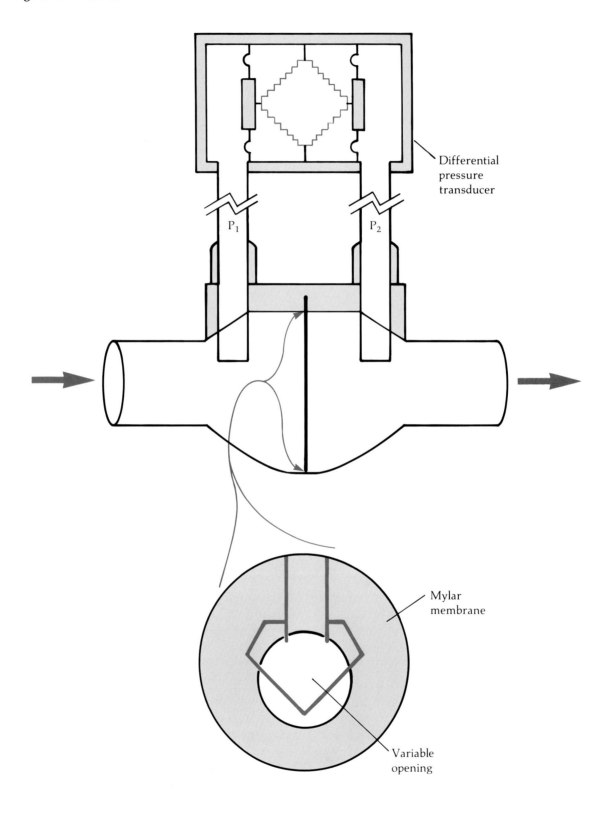

Differential
pressure
transducer

P_1

P_2

Mylar
membrane

Variable
opening

Figure 2.9— Bird flow transducer.

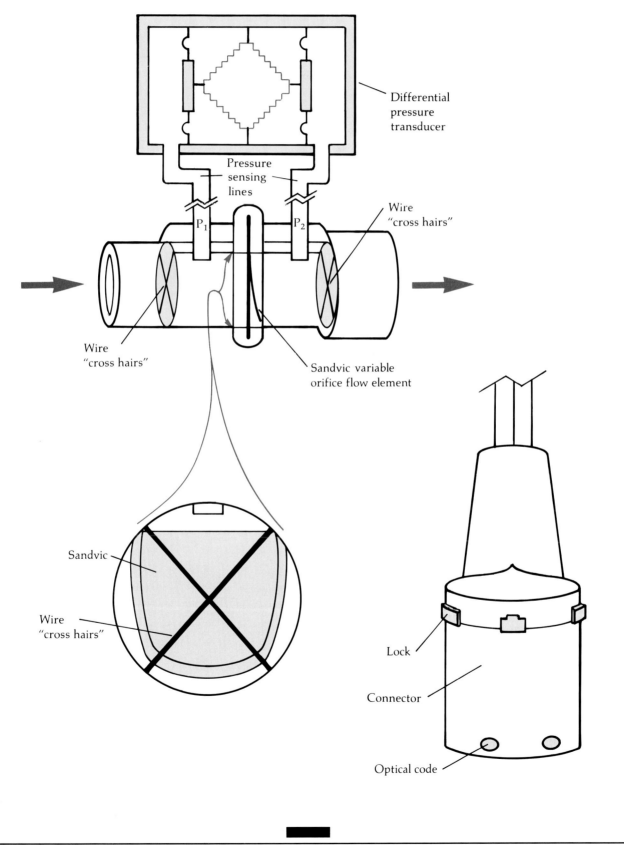

Figure 2.10— The static paramagnetic oxygen analyzer.

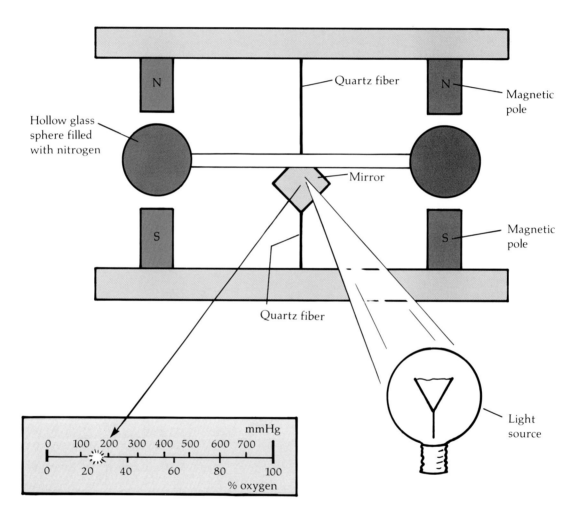

flow rates can contribute to inaccurate results, this particular analyzer is rarely used in patient care.

2.4.2 Dynamic or Magneto-Acoustic Paramagnetic Analyzer

Although technically an invasive device, the O_2 analyzer in the Datex AGM-13 Capnomac™ is a modern adaptation of the paramagnetic principle. Two gases, the gas to be measured and the reference gas (usually room air), are drawn at a rate of 200 ml/min. into the gap between the poles of a strong electromagnetic field. As the current to the electromagnet switches cyclically on and off, a pressure signal proportional to the O_2 content difference between the two gases is generated. The signal is picked up with a differential pressure transducer (Figure 2.11).

Clinical considerations: The principle advantages of this type of cell are the fast response time of 150 milliseconds or greater, the capability for breath-to-breath measurement, and the capability for differential analysis.[7] The cell is somewhat sensitive to humidity and vibration, but insensitive to light, temperature variations, patient movement, and poor peripheral perfusion. With the Datex product, airway O_2 measurement including inspired oxygen (FiO_2), end-tidal oxygen (ETO_2), and oxygrams are possible.[8] Oxygrams are the changing graphic representation of the inspired and expired O_2 waveforms during the respiratory cycle. According to the manufacturer, the inspired/end-tidal O_2 difference (FiO_2-ETO_2) is more sensitive than end-tidal oxygen for the determination of hypoventilation. Because of the high sampling rate of 200 ml/min, this device is not suitable for use in small pediatric and neonatal patients.

2.4.3 Thermal Conductivity Analyzer

Oxygen molecules have the ability to carry and, therefore, dissipate heat. Using this principle of thermal conductivity, O_2 analyzers measure the concentration of O_2 in a gas sample by observing the changes in electrical resistance. Remember that the conductivity of a wire is proportional to the temperature of the wire. To measure the cooling effect of the O_2 molecules, an electrical circuit of comparative resistances, commonly called a Wheatstone bridge, is used (Figure 2.12). The circuit consists of two cells. The sample cell (Cell 1 or C_1) and the reference cell (Cell 2 or C_2).

Cell 2 is open to the atmosphere. If room air enters into Cell 1, the cooling effect in the two cells is identical, as is the current through ABD as compared to the current through ACD (Figure 2.12). If a sample of gas with a higher concentration of O_2 is introduced into C_1, the cooling effect will be higher and the current will be greater with respect to C_2. This potential difference, measured by the galvanometer, is proportional to the number of O_2 molecules cooling the resistance wire in C_1.

Clinical considerations: As with the paramagnetic O_2 analyzers, the thermal conductivity type is relatively labor intensive and, therefore, designed for intermittent sampling. Gas flow and H_2O vapor increase the cooling effect of the resistance wires and result in higher readings. Additionally, other gases, such as CO_2, have similar thermal conductivity properties and can interfere with the cooling effect of O_2 molecules.

Figure 2.11— Dynamic paramagnetic analyzer.

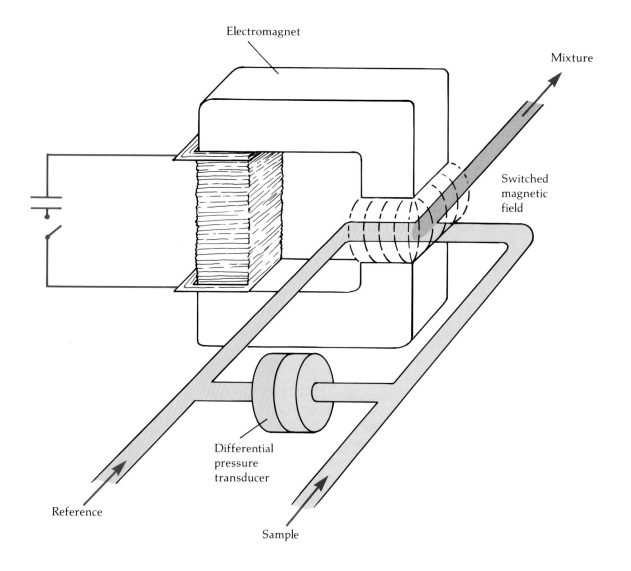

Electromagnet

Mixture

Switched
magnetic
field

Differential
pressure
transducer

Reference

Sample

2.4.4   Electrochemical Sensors

The O_2 sensors commonly used for routine measurements of inspiratory O_2 in patient ventilator circuits are based on electrochemical methods. The two major types of electrochemical O_2 sensors are the polarographic type and the galvanic or fuel cell type. The basic electrochemical cell contains two electrodes immersed in an electrolyte. The gas sample electrolytically reacts at the electrode-electrolyte interface and, depending on the configuration of the cell, generates a current or voltage proportional to the gas concentration. The electrochemical sensors are mainstream type sensors because no sampling system is required. The main advantage of these sensors is their simplicity and low cost. The main disadvantage is that they have a limited lifespan.

If only a one-point calibration is performed, a one-point calibration with 100% O_2 is better than a one-point calibration with room air (21%). A two-point calibration using room air and 100% O_2 is best since it determines the true linearity or characteristic curve of the sensor. A significant deviation from linearity indicates that the sensor is nearing the end of its useful life and probably should be discarded. Many of the newer sensors require calibration only once per day although some manufacturers still recommend a recalibration every 8 hours.

Since the sensor measures the partial pressure (not the percentage) of O_2, changes in the barometric pressure alter the reading even if the percentage of O_2 in the sample remains constant. The partial pressure of oxygen (P_{O_2}) is equal to the percent of oxygen (%O_2) times the pressure at which the sample is measured:

$$P_{O_2} \;=\; (\% \, O_2) \;\; (\text{mm Hg or cm } H_2O) \qquad \textbf{Equation 2.1}$$

If the barometric pressure at sea level is 760 mm Hg (1034 cm H_2O) and dry air contains 21% O_2, then:

$$
\begin{aligned}
P_{O_2} \;&=\; (21\%) \;\; (760 \text{ mm Hg or } 1034 \text{ cm } H_2O) \quad \textbf{Equation 2.2} \\
&=\; 160 \text{ mm Hg or } 217 \text{ cm } H_2O
\end{aligned}
$$

The presence of humidity in the sample gas decreases the actual concentration of O_2 because H_2O vapor exerts its own pressure. If 100% O_2 is saturated with H_2O vapor, the actual concentration of O_2 drops from 100% to 96% to 97%. Therefore, an analyzer calibrated in dry gas will display a slightly lower reading in a humidified gas. If the analyzer sensor is calibrated on the dry side of the ventilator circuit before the humidifier, the reading will be slightly higher than the actual percentage of O_2 delivered to the patient because humidity introduced after the O_2 sensor dilutes the gas mixture after it has been measured. For this reason, the analyzer/monitor should never be calibrated in an atmosphere saturated with H_2O vapor. Additionally, excessive condensation on the semipermeable membrane can cause a mechanical obstruction for the diffusion of O_2 through the membrane. If used in a high humidity environment, O_2 analyzer sensors should be placed in the independent position so that condensation drains away from the surface of the membrane.

The effects of temperature on the O_2 sensor are quite small. But when added to the effects of H_2O vapor and pressure, the total effect can be quite significant. Most modern sensors incorporate a thermistor as part of the cell so that variations due to temperature changes are minimized.

Figure 2.12— Thermal conductivity analyzer.

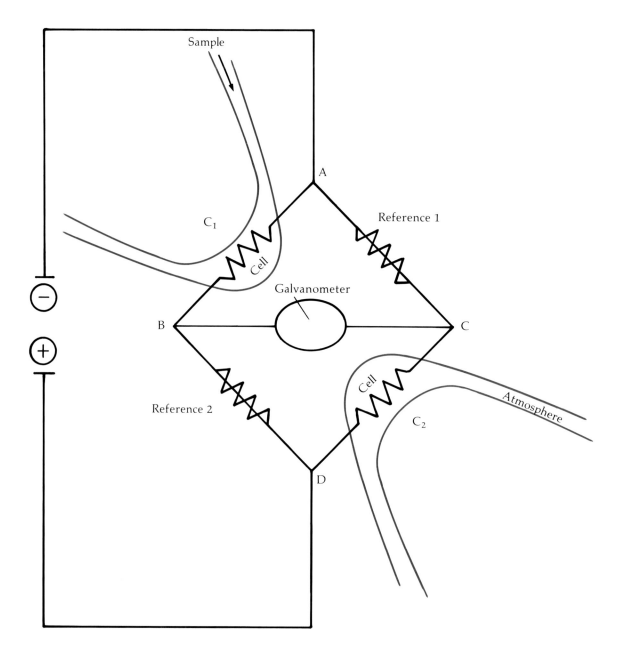

In summary, to correct the displayed O_2 percentage for humidity and system pressure, use the following equation:

$$\%O_2 \text{ (corrected)} = \%O_2 \text{ (displayed)} \times \text{(ambient pressure - } H_2O \text{ vapor pressure at the system temperature/mean system pressure)}$$

The mean system pressure is the ambient pressure plus the mean pressure due to the ventilator. If the displayed O_2 percentage is 90%, the ambient pressure is 1034 cm H_2O, the vapor pressure of H_2O at 37 degrees centigrade is 64 cm H_2O, and the mean system pressure is 10 cm H_2O, then:

$$\%O_2 \text{ (corrected)} = (90\%) \ (1034 - 64/1034 + 10)$$
or $$\%O_2 \text{ (corrected)} = (90\%) \cdot (970 \text{ cm } H_2O/1044 \text{ cm } H_2O)$$
or $$\%O_2 \text{ (corrected)} = 83.6\%$$

As can be seen from this example, it is important to understand the effects of vapor pressure and system pressure on the displayed concentration of O_2.

Since the effects of various other gases vary somewhat with the manufacturer of the cell in use, it is best to consult the specifications for the particular cell. Gases with an equal to or less than 1% O_2 error are nitrogen, helium, and nitrous oxide to 80%, and CO_2 to 12%. Common anesthetics such as isoflurane, methoxyflurane, and halothane can introduce up to a 2% O_2 error but do not damage the performance of the O_2 sensor.

2.4.4.1 **Polarographic Sensor**

The polarographic cell, which is an electrochemical cell, was invented by Leland C. Clark in 1954 and is often called the Clark electrode.[9] Polarographic analysis uses the ability of O_2 to chemically react with H_2O in the presence of electrons (e^-) to produce hydroxyl (OH^-) ions. This electrochemical reaction requires a constant externally applied voltage of −0.6 volts which supplies electrons via a cathode of gold (Au) or platinum (Pt) (Figure 2.13). Oxygen is reduced at the cathode:

Chemical Reaction #1: $\qquad O_2 + 2H_2O + 4e^- \longleftrightarrow 4OH^-$

The resulting hydroxyl ions migrate to and react with the silver (Ag) anode and release their charge. Oxidation occurs at the anode:

Chemical Reaction #2: $\qquad 4OH^- + 4Ag \longleftrightarrow 2Ag_2O + 2H_2O + 4e^-$

The magnitude of the resulting current between the anode and the cathode, measured by an ammeter, is directly proportional to the number of O_2 molecules.

The electrochemical cells using the polarographic principle are constructed so that the anode and cathode are surrounded by an electrolyte of potassium chloride and lie in close proximity to an O_2^- permeable membrane constructed of teflon or polypropylene. As O_2 molecules traverse the membrane, they combine with H_2O and electrons to form hydroxyl ions. The hydroxyl ions migrate to the Ag/AgCl anode, react with the silver, and release the electrons. The electron flow is measured by the ammeter and converted on a scale of O_2 concentration.

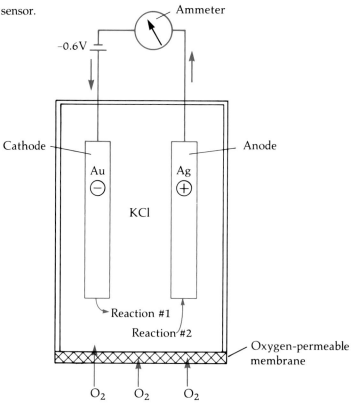

Figure 2.13— Polarographic sensor.

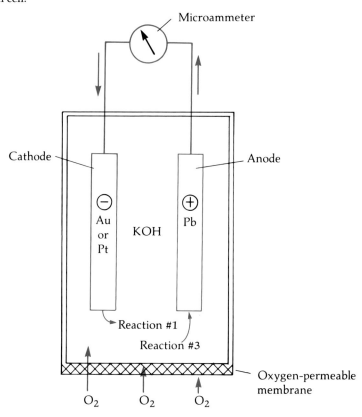

Figure 2.14— Galvanic/fuel cell.

Clinical considerations: The response time of the cell depends on the thickness of the membrane.[10] A very thin membrane may be responsive enough to permit breath-to-breath measurements. Typically, the cells are given a one-year warranty by the manufacturer.

2.4.4.2 Galvanic or Fuel Cell Sensor

Unlike the polarographic cell, which must have a constant voltage to polarize the electrode, another electrochemical cell—the galvanic or fuel cell—produces electrical energy without an external electrical source.[11] The construction of the galvanic cell resembles the polarographic type (Figure 2.14). The cathode is gold or platinum, the anode is lead or copper, and the electrolyte is usually potassium hydroxide.

As O_2 molecules diffuse through the O_2^- permeable membrane of the cell, they chemically react with the H_2O in the electrolyte to form hydroxyl ions. Oxygen is consumed to produce a current (See Chemical Reaction #1 above). The hydroxyl ions migrate to the lead (Pb) anode, react with it, and produce electrons. As in the polarographic type, the electrolyte facilitates the ionic migration:

Chemical Reaction #3: $4OH^- + Pb \longleftrightarrow PbO_2 + 2H_2O + 4e^-$

The current flow resulting from this reaction is measured by a microammeter and displayed as a percentage of O_2. The rate of this reaction is temperature dependent. Newer galvanic O_2 sensors have thermistors incorporated in the sensor to correct the current flow to compensate for variations in temperature.

Clinical considerations: The typical galvanic cell is somewhat slower than the polarographic cell.[12,13] The life expectancy of the galvanic fuel cells varies with the manufacturer. Most cells have a warranty of one year from the date of purchase. The C-l type cell will last 240,000 hours, while the C-2 cell will last only 100,000 hours. This means that the higher the concentration of O_2 the cell is exposed to, the shorter its life. If a typical value is 200,000 hours, the cell will last about three months in 100% O_2 and about 15 months in room air. Because the cell begins to deteriorate as soon as it is exposed to O_2, most cells are packaged in nitrogen.

2.5 Capnography

Capnography is the graphic representation, as well as the interpretation, of the waveform of the changing concentration of CO_2 during the entire respiratory cycle.[8] Capnography is based on the fact that all mammalian cells have in common the ability to obtain energy for their specific functions by using O_2 to burn glucose to their end products of CO_2 and H_2O. For CO_2 to be detected, metabolism must occur in the cell with the production of CO_2, CO_2 must be transported from the cell to the lung by the circulation, and the CO_2 must be eliminated by diffusion into the alveoli and through the airways by ventilation. In the breathing cycle the CO_2-rich gases of expiration are exchanged for fresh non-CO_2-containing gases on the inspiratory phase, producing the characteristic CO_2 waveform.

The two types of CO_2 monitors currently in use today are the mainstream and sidestream types. The detector in the mainstream monitor attaches to the airway adapter connected to the endotracheal tube and is an integral part of the airway. The sidestream type, which is typically invasive, samples the stream of gas and conducts the sample to the infrared optical bench in the monitor. Capnography and capnometry continue to be underused and misunderstood technologies today. For an excellent discussion of the operation and application of these two types of capnometers, please refer to Section 6.0, Capnography and Gas Monitoring, in this volume.

2.6   *Humidity Determination*

Although H_2O vapor is one of the most common constituents in the humidified gas delivered by modern ventilators, the application of humidity sensors to the ventilator circuit has not been developed. It has been assumed that the delivered gas, as it passes through a heated humidifier, becomes 100% saturated. Evidence for this assumption is that H_2O "rains out" in the ventilator tubing. But questions remain: is the heated, humidified gas 100% saturated throughout the ventilator assisted breathing cycle? And, does it make a clinical difference? In neonates and long-term ventilator patients, under-humidified gas dries the normal respiratory secretions and creates another set of difficulties such as infection and airway collapse. Further research is needed in the area of humidity determination.[14] Halogenated polymeric sensors or surface acoustic wave technology microsensors may soon be adapted to the airway environment for the detection and measurement of humidity.[15]

2.7   *Waveform and Graphic Analysis*

With the incorporation of microprocessors in mechanical ventilators and patient monitors, the clinician has many types of displays available for medical information. One difficulty for the clinician is the separation of the parameters of the mechanical ventilator from those of the spontaneously breathing patient. This situation occurs with a sporadically breathing patient who needs support from a mechanical ventilator while recovering from open heart surgery. Since most of the modern ventilators have the O_2 sensors and differential pressure and flow transducers incorporated within the ventilator for protection, one must question the accuracy of these devices when considering the parameters necessary for adequate monitoring of the patient. For example, can the ventilator performance be accurately differentiated from the patient response to a specific volume? This can become a significant issue when the distance from the ventilator outlet to the patient "Y" can exceed four feet in length. When flow transducers located close to the patient "Y" generate a differential pressure, will that pressure have the accuracy necessary for a proper clinical picture when interpreted up to four feet away? These and many other factors must be considered in the continuing development of biosensor technology as it applies to the patient airway.

For a well written analysis on flow, pressure, and volume monitoring in the mechanically ventilated and the spontaneously breathing patient, refer to "Graphical Analysis of Flow, Pressure, and Volume During Mechanical Ventilation" by Macintyre, Bear Medical Systems, 1991.[16] Another excellent publication on this subject is "Waveforms, The Graphical Presentation of Ventilatory Data" by the Puritan Bennett Corporation, 1990.[17]

2.8   *Future Directions*

The key words in any discussion of the future directions of airway monitoring must include the words noninvasive and reusable. Today's care providers using body substance isolation techniques are faced with the tasks of protecting themselves from the patients, the patients from the care providers, and the patients from each other. By providing patients with sterile reusable ventilator circuits, the possibility of nosocomial contamination is virtually eliminated. Institutions gain economically when they use reusable materials. Those institutions that choose disposable ventilator circuits, for example, are using "medically clean," not sterile, circuits. They must also pay for disposing of the medical waste. The long-term cost of disposables is as much a detriment to the institution as it is to the ecology.

A biotechnological sensor that is reusable and an integral part of the ventilator circuit can also be noninvasive. A sensor can be part of the ventilator circuit but, also, can sample the gas flowing through the circuit. A side-stream capnometer, for example, "invades" the circuit and, therefore, may contaminate the transmission as well as contribute to the inaccuracy of downstream pressure, flow, and volume measurements.

2.8.1 The Expansion of Noninvasive Biotechnology Sensors

Optical technology or fiberoptics can convey, send, and receive different types of light across the airway and to a remote monitor.[18-21] For example, shielded fiberoptics can convey the infrared light used by some capnometers and pulse oximeters. The total weight of the airway sensor can be reduced and yet maintain a high degree of accuracy since the sensor is placed as close to the patient as possible. Optical technology and fiberoptics can also transmit information rapidly and accurately without any dampening of the signal over great distances. The optical fiber thermometer currently in use in some areas of anesthesiology and the practice of family medicine can be incorporated into the inspiratory and expiratory limbs of the airway tubing. The actual temperature of the delivered gas and the temperature differential between the inspired and expired gases can be determined.

Chemical sensors that change colors in the presence of different variables such as CO_2 (like the Fenum FEF® device) and relative humidity are being refined and expanded to respond to the wide variety of conditions encountered at the airway in the mechanically ventilated or spontaneously breathing patient. Invasive chemical sensors, such as those presently in use and under development, are limited by the site life. For example, the life of a radial artery cannula site in most clinical situations is 48 hours. This is very expensive technology fraught with hazards, such as infection potential, clot formation, and occlusion, which can be avoided by using noninvasive technologies.

Moisture or relative humidity sensors can be incorporated in the airway so that the true relative humidity can be determined on the inspiratory side as well as the expiratory limb of the ventilator circuit. Through microprocessors, the true effect of humidity can correct the pressure, flow, volume, F_IO_2, F_EO_2, and $ETCO_2$ readings. The result of these calculations can produce a more accurate representation of the true clinical picture of the patient.

Laser-doppler anemometer sensors are being developed to provide a real-time integration of flow and volume measurements.[22]

Further developments in noninvasive breath-by-breath inspired and expired O_2 determination can have significant ramifications for the clinician, in particular the ability to accurately determine the O_2 consumption and, therefore, the respiratory quotient and nutritional requirements of the intensive care patient.[23] Currently, the accuracy of these measurements is directly proportional to the accuracy of the O_2 analyzer. Therefore, the application of these devices in their current configurations has not been well accepted by the clinician.

2.8.2 Quick and Accurate (Intuitive) Medical Graphics

Because of the capabilities and complexities of modern biotechnological sensors, microprocessors, and computers, care providers and decision makers often do not completely comprehend the numbers, waveforms, and data from these instruments. The graphic displays available to the clinician are numerous and extremely varied. They include analog displays with traditional bar graphs and monitored "out-of-limits" markers, polygon displays presenting key-monitored variables, numeric displays, graphic trend displays, digital trend displays, loops, waveform displays, and many other combinations and permutations. With the exception of the polygons, most of these displays are "flat" or typical X- and Y- axis presentations. Quick and accurate interpretation of this myriad of information is difficult or lacking because it is not intuitive.

When five critical ventilation variables from the respiratory care flow sheet (FiO_2, respiratory rate, tidal volume, spontaneous respiratory rate, and spontaneous tidal volume) are displayed as graphic representations or icons instead of horizontal tabular bands of numbers, a clinician briefly introduced to the concept can make clinical decisions faster than when using tabular data. This does not suggest that graphic representations result in faster decisions. The graphic representation must be easy to learn, intuitively pleasing, and valuable in the interpretation of clinical data.

Because the human brain can discriminate minute differences in graphic characters more rapidly and accurately than it can interpret numbers, intuitive graphics permit the rapid scanning of large amounts of information. Further development of intuitive graphic representations for other disciplines such as cardiac monitoring and pharmacology may fundamentally alter human information processing in data intensive situations that require decision making.[24,25]

3.0 PULSE OXIMETRY

Pulse oximeters have evolved from physiologic monitoring curiosities to common patient monitoring devices. New pulse oximetry technology couples spectrophotometry with pulse waveform monitoring and permits clinicians to continuously assess arterial O_2 saturation in operating rooms, in intensive care units, during sleep studies (polysomnography), and at the bedside. Portable pulse oximeters and recorders have also become popular monitoring devices during emergency medical transport and outpatient assessment of gas exchange. Advantages to pulse oximeters, other than their noninvasiveness, include their well-documented accuracy, ease of application, and good patient tolerance.

Continuous pulse oximetric monitoring of arterial oxygenation can detect intermittent or chronic disruptions in gas exchange that may not be detected by random arterial blood sampling and analysis. Also, pulse oximeter measurements of O_2 saturation do not carry the risk of morbidity and mortality associated with invasive arterial blood sampling. Another value of continuous monitoring is the ability to quantitatively determine the amount of time spent at any given level of arterial O_2 saturation.[26] This information can then be used to monitor the progression of gas exchange impairment or to evaluate the effectiveness of therapeutic interventions. With such widespread application of pulse oximetry technology, comprehension of the operating principles and the practical limitations of use can aid clinicians. This section describes the fundamental principles used in pulse oximetry technology to acquaint clinicians with environmental and physiological conditions that can affect their use.

3.1 An Overview of the Development of Pulse Oximetry

Development of noninvasive spectrophotometric techniques to monitor O_2 saturation began during World War II.[27] The development of high altitude aircraft created a need for pilots to be noninvasively monitored for any physiological changes induced by extreme altitude. In response to this need, the first functional noninvasive spectrophotometer was developed by 1942. Its inventor, Glen Millikan, named this new device the "oximeter" (Figure 3.1).[28] By using two optical filters to transmit light through the pinna of the ear, the oximeter measured the color of the hemoglobin molecule. From the color, the oximeter calculated total hemoglobin saturation.

Other than some minor changes to Millikan's oximeter, noninvasive oximetric technology research remained essentially dormant until the introduction of the ear oximeter in 1975. This oximeter used fiberoptic cables to transmit light to a housing strapped to the pinna of the subject's ear. The cable housing had a heating element to warm the monitoring site and cause nearby arterioles to dilate. Since the warmed monitoring site was effectively arterialized, the ear oximeter essentially measured the O_2 saturation of arterial blood. The ear oximeter used eight light wavelengths to differentiate oxyhemoglobin from reduced hemoglobin, skin, tissue, and dyshemoglobins, a significant improvement over Millikan's oximeter, which could not make such distinctions.

While the ear oximeter received acclaim as a research tool, it never gained widespread acceptance for clinical applications due to its impractical size, cumbersome headgear, and high cost. Due to the limitations of ear oximetry, noninvasive monitoring of O_2 saturation was used primarily for research rather than clinical purposes. However, with the advent of light-emitting diodes (LEDs), photodetectors, and miniaturized amplifiers, Japanese researchers developed the first "pulse oximeters". This low cost, state-of-the-art, noninvasive monitoring technique innovatively coupled spectrophotometry (which measures O_2 bound to hemoglobin) with photoplethysmography (which measures arterial pulsations). The combination of these principles resulted in an instrument that could differentiate arterial from venous blood to selectively measure arterial O_2 saturation with only two light wavelengths instead of the eight required by the ear oximeter.

3.2 Fundamentals in Spectrophotometry and Photoplethysmography

To noninvasively measure arterial O_2 saturation, pulse oximeters combine two techniques of light transmission and reception: spectrophotometry and photoplethysmography.

Figure 3.1— Early version of an ear oximeter.

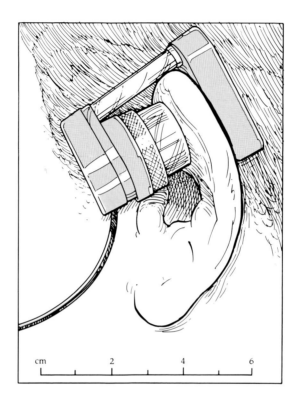

Figure 3.2— Oxyhemoglobin and deoxyhemoglobin absorption (extinction) characteristics.

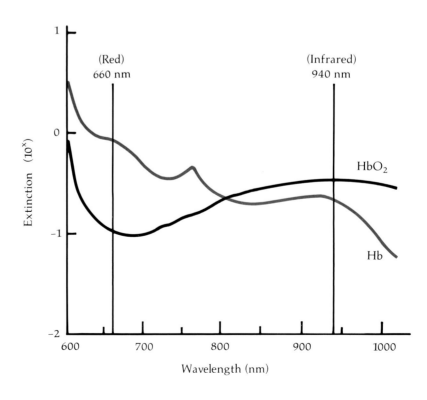

Spectrophotometry determines the percentage of oxygenated hemoglobin in the blood while photoplethysmography differentiates arterial from venous blood.[29,30]

Spectrophotometers measure hemoglobin saturation since the color and optical density of the hemoglobin molecule changes according to the amount of O_2 bound to it.[31] Oxygenated hemoglobin appears bright red while deoxygenated hemoglobin is dark blue. Therefore, each species of hemoglobin has its own light absorption characteristics.[31,32] Figure 3.2 shows that the largest difference in absorption characteristics between oxygenated hemoglobin and deoxygenated hemoglobin occurs near the 660-nanometer (nm) range, which is the frequency of red light. Therefore, when a red light (near 660 nm) is transmitted through well-oxygenated, bright red blood, a significant amount of the light passes through the hemoglobin. On the other hand, if the blood is deoxygenated and dark, much less light is able to pass through the hemoglobin.

In addition to the red light, pulse oximetry uses a second light wavelength to calculate O_2 saturation. This wavelength is called isobestic, meaning that oxygenated, as well as deoxygenated, hemoglobin will absorb about the same amount of it.[33] Figure 3.2 illustrates that the isobestic, or crossover, point in light absorption between oxygenated hemoglobin and deoxygenated hemoglobin is near 805 nm, which is in the infrared range. Also in Figure 3.2, two vertical lines, one at 660 nm and one at 940 nm, indicate the light wavelengths produced by currently available LEDs.

Red light transmission through blood is dependant upon hemoglobin saturation and infrared light is not. Therefore, a ratio between the intensity of the transmitted-to-received red and infrared light can be calculated. Figure 3.3, a block diagram of a pulse oximeter front end, illustrates the various components that produce and measure red and infrared lights. It is the ratio of red to infrared light that the oximeter uses to derive a value of O_2 saturation. Figure 3.4 presents red to infrared light ratios and their corresponding values of O_2 saturation. To determine these values of O_2 saturation from the ratios of red and infrared light wavelengths, an empirical calibration curve is developed through studies in healthy human subjects.

To develop a calibration curve, one protocol requires human subjects to have an in-dwelling arterial catheter inserted. Then the sensor of the pulse oximeter being tested is attached to a well-perfused monitoring site (usually a finger or an ear). While his or her fractional inspired O_2 concentration is closely monitored (either with mass spectroscopy or other types of monitoring devices), the subject breathes an isocapnic, hypoxic gas mixture to lower their arterial O_2 saturation to a predetermined level.[34] Serial blood samples drawn from the indwelling catheter are analyzed for arterial O_2 saturation by co-oximetry and are correlated with simultaneous pulse oximeter values of red and infrared lights. The value of O_2 saturation (as measured by the co-oximeter from the blood sample) is then assigned to the ratio of red to infrared light received by the pulse oximeter. This procedure is repeated at many different levels of O_2 saturation in a series of subjects until a calibration curve is generated. By performing studies on numerous subjects, the oximeter can then be empirically validated.

Photoplethysmography uses light reflectance or light transmission through vascular tissue to measure arterial pressure waveforms generated by the cardiac cycle. In turn, noninvasive relative estimates of arterial blood flow, blood pressure, and tissue perfusion can also be obtained. The basic principle of photoplethysmography is: if a constant amount of light is transmitted through a pulsating vascular bed, more light is transmitted through the bed when the arterioles are nearly empty (cardiac diastole) than when the arterioles are mostly full (cardiac systole).[35]

Figure 3.3— Block diagram of a pulse oximetry amplifier.

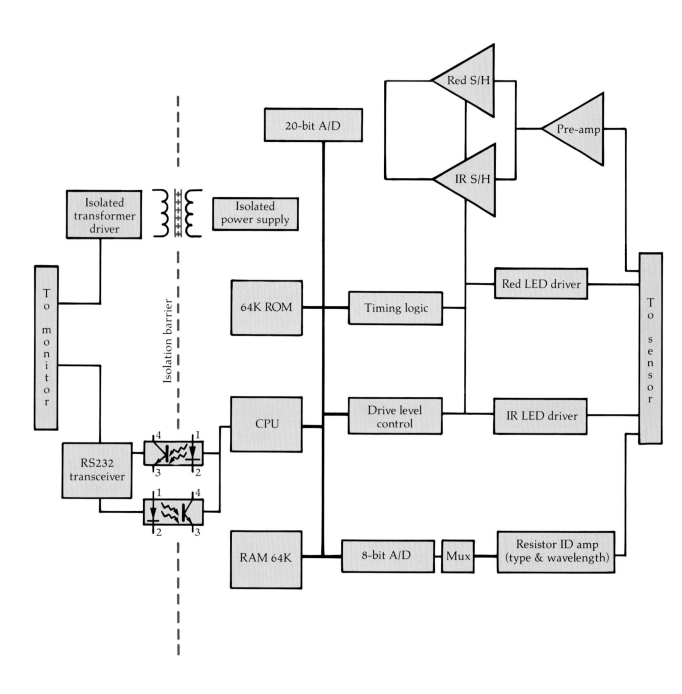

The filling and emptying of the arterioles affect the pathlength of the transmitted light which causes the received light's intensity to fluctuate. The fluctuating part of the received light's intensity is defined as the alternating current (AC) signal. Additionally, other potential modifiers of the transmitted light exist, such as tissue, venous blood, as well as a portion of the arterial blood (Figure 3.5). However, since these substances absorb a constant amount of the transmitted light, their influence upon the transmission and reception of the light signal is essentially static. This static portion of the signal is called the direct current (DC) signal. By isolating the pulsatile, or AC, portion of the received light and spectrophotometrically measuring O_2 bound to hemoglobin during that time, this information has been shown to correlate better with arterial O_2 saturation.

3.3   *Pulse Oximeter Sensor Technology*

After the first pulse oximeters were built, sensor technology played an important role in the transition of pulse oximetry technology from research laboratories to a clinical setting. The typical pulse oximeter sensor configuration is one or two red LEDs and an infrared LED, all of which are located on one side of the monitoring site. A photoreceiver is positioned on the opposite side of the monitoring site, directly opposing the LEDs. The red and infrared LEDs function to transmit red and infrared light, while the photoreceiver measures their intensity on the opposite side of the monitoring site. These types of sensors in which light is transmitted by LEDs and received by a photoreceiver are called transmittance sensors.

The primary functional requirement for transmittance sensors is that the monitoring site should not be so thick as to prevent transmission of light through it. This often limits sensor sites to either fingers, ears, or toes. To overcome this limitation, a new generation of reflectance sensors have recently become available.[36] Reflectance oximetry transmits light into a pulsatile vascular bed, which is then reflected back to the photoreceiver positioned next to the LEDs. Since this single-sided sensor can be placed virtually anywhere on the body, forehead sensor placement could overcome the problem of peripheral extremity vasoconstriction during surgery, a condition that decreases distal pulse pressures, thereby creating unstable saturation values when using a finger sensor. Patients with burns or edema would also benefit from a reflectance sensor not restricted to finger or ear placement.

While reflectance sensors use backscattered rather than transmitted light, the signal analysis is similar to that of transmittance pulse sensors. However, the pulse oximeter has a smaller amplitude signal to work with. Consequently, it must increase the gain of the signal reception to bring the pulse waveform signal into a usable range. This, in turn, can produce an unstable system that may be overly sensitive to motion. However, if reflectance oximetry is used in anesthetized or immobile patients, its ease of sensor placement may outweigh its sensitivity to motion artifact.

3.4   *Technical Limitations of Pulse Oximetry*

As previously described, pulse oximeters derive values of O_2 saturation from a ratio of transmitted-to-received red and infrared light. While the primary modifier of this red-to-infrared ratio is the color of the hemoglobin molecule (of which methemoglobin and

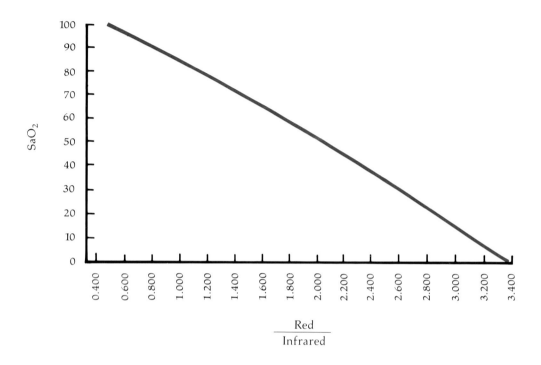

Figure 3.4— Red-to-infrared light ratios with their corresponding values of arterial oxygen saturation.

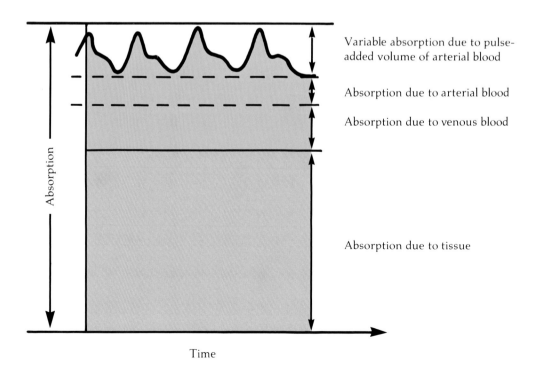

Figure 3.5— Tissue composite shows dynamic and static components affecting light absorption.

Variable absorption due to pulse-added volume of arterial blood

Absorption due to arterial blood

Absorption due to venous blood

Absorption due to tissue

carboxyhemoglobin are also modifiers of the red-to-infrared ratios) dyshemoglobins are forms of hemoglobin that do not bind O_2 but do affect the color of the hemoglobin molecule.

Since four distinct species of hemoglobin exist in the blood: reduced hemoglobin, oxyhemoglobin, methemoglobin, and carboxyhemoglobin, four separate light wavelengths are required to differentiate one from the other. Once each type of hemoglobin is identified, the ratio of oxyhemoglobin to total hemoglobin can be calculated. This ratio is termed *fractional* O_2 saturation. Fractional O_2 saturation is the value produced by co-oximeters, devices that produce in vitro measurements of O_2 saturation.

As Figure 3.6 illustrates, deoxyhemoglobin and methemoglobin absorb similar amounts of red light at a wavelength near 660 nm. Also, carboxyhemoglobin and oxyhemoglobin have almost identical absorption characteristics at 660 nm. Consequently, pulse oximeters that use a red light frequency near 660 nm cannot differentiate methemoglobin from deoxyhemoglobin, nor can they differentiate oxyhemoglobin from carboxyhemoglobin.[37] Therefore, the value that pulse oximeters display as percent O_2 saturation is actually a sum of the four hemoglobin species and is termed *functional* saturation (% SaO_2 func).

Figure 3.6— Hemoglobin extinction curves of deoxyhemoglobin, oxyhemoglobin, carboxyhemoglobin, and methemoglobin.

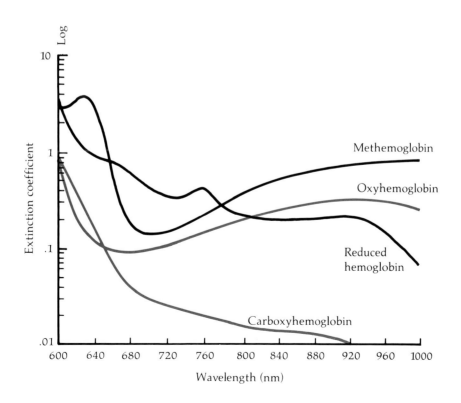

$$\%\text{SaO}_2 \text{ func} = \frac{\text{SaO}_2 \text{ frac} \times 100}{100 - (\%\text{COHb} + \%\text{MetHb})}$$

Equation 3.1

where $\%\text{SaO}_2$ frac   =   fractional O_2 saturation

                         $\%\text{COHb}$ =   percent carboxyhemoglobin

                         $\%\text{MetHb}$ =   percent methemoglobin.

Fortunately, the percentage of carboxyhemoglobin and methemoglobin in healthy, nonsmoking subjects is relatively small so their presence does not significantly alter the accuracy of pulse oximeters. However, as described below, there are occasions when excessive amounts of dyshemoglobins can markedly affect a pulse oximeter's ability to accurately measure O_2 saturation.

Carbon monoxide binds with hemoglobin more readily than does O_2. In cases of CO poisoning, the presence of carboxyhemoglobin causes the arterial blood to become bright red.[38] The pulse oximeter cannot differentiate carboxyhemoglobin from oxyhemoglobin since both have similar light absorption characteristics near 660 nm. This peculiarity associated with CO poisoning and hemoglobin coloring could prove potentially lethal if pulse oximetry alone is used as a method of assessing oxygenation. In cases of smoke inhalation or suspected CO poisoning, assessment of an invasive arterial blood sample by co-oximetry is necessary to measure carboxyhemoglobin.

In the light wavelength range near 660 nm, methemoglobin has absorption characteristics similar to deoxyhemoglobin. Consequently, pulse oximetry cannot discern methemoglobin from deoxyhemoglobin. Certain clinical conditions in which excess methemoglobin exists may cause the pulse oximeter to falsely display low values of O_2 saturation.[39]

Radiographic dyes injected into a patient will also affect the accuracy of pulse oximeters.[40,41] Since most radiographic dyes are either methyl blue or green, a prominent amount of blue dye in the arterial blood can be misinterpreted by the oximeter as being deoxyhemoglobin. These effects of intravascular dyes are transient, but if they are unrecognized, it may lead to erroneous clinical decisions.

In anemic states, whether transiently induced during open heart surgery by thermodilution or pathologically induced by chronic renal failure, an increased chance of pulse oximeter error exists. In the anemic normoxic patient, pulse oximetry appears to be fairly accurate.[40,41] However, in the patient suspected of being hypoxic, pulse oximetry values should be validated by invasive arterial blood samples. The basis of concern, shown in theoretical models but not yet duplicated in a clinical setting, is that the pulse oximeter algorithm is programmed to use a light intensity strong enough to transmit through a certain thickness of tissue, and thus expects the red light to be scattered by a predetermined amount of red blood cells in any given area.[42] The pulse oximeter can increase or decrease its light transmission intensity to compensate for tissue thickness and light scattering. However, if due to an anemic condition, the light may not be scattered to the degree expected, too much of the transmitted red light will reach the photoreceiver, potentially creating a falsely high value of O_2 saturation.

Dark skin pigmentation is associated with greater degrees of error in pulse oximetry measurements.[43,44] One possible mechanism of the measurement error is a shunting of the red and infrared light around the periphery of the monitoring site. Since light follows the path of least resistance, in darkly pigmented people a portion of the transmitted light may travel subcutaneously from the LEDs to the photoreceiver. If the shunted light that reaches the photoreceiver has assumed low grade AC characteristics, the ratio of red to infrared light could potentially be affected. Since subcutaneously shunted light is never exposed to a vascular bed, its intensity is not modulated by the color of the hemoglobin or by the pulsating arterioles. Therefore, the red-to-infrared ratios of shunted light will be different from the red-to-infrared ratios from transmitted and received lights. When shunted and unshunted red and infrared light reach the photosensor, their effect upon each other may produce erroneous values of O_2 saturation.

Alternatively, if shunted light does not develop AC characteristics its presence is still noted by the photoreceiver as electrical noise. This increased noise-to-signal ratio also can potentially cause a display of erroneous values of O_2 saturation.

Pulse oximeter sensors have separate LEDs to transmit red and infrared light. However, the sensor only has one photoreceiver to measure each light. To assess each light independently, the pulse oximeter first flashes on the red LED and the photoreceiver measures its intensity after it has passed through the monitoring site. It then turns the red LED off. Next, the infrared LED is switched on and the photoreceiver measures its intensity after it has passed through the monitoring site. The infrared LED is then switched off. Finally, both LEDs are off and the photoreceiver measures the ambient light intensity which is subtracted from the values of red and infrared light. This sequence occurs several hundred times per second.

Intense light from fluorescent lamps, operating room lights, and infrared heat lamps have been reported to interfere with pulse oximeter performance.[45,46] External infrared light sources may increase the intensity of the infrared signal measured by the sensor's photoreceiver. Consequently, this may lower both the displayed heart rate and O_2 saturation. While these events may not appear in a readily reproducible fashion, they should be considered when using a pulse oximeter sensor.

3.5 Additional Factors That Affect Pulse Oximeter Accuracy

3.5.1 Motion Artifact

When a pulse oximeter sensor is on a monitoring site that is subject to motion, the intermittent contact of the sensor with the skin can mechanically modulate the pathlength of the transmitted light. In turn, the ratios of red to infrared light are no longer modulated by the color of the hemoglobin molecule or by the pulsating vascular bed. If the motion is repetitive or persistent, signals of similar amplitude are received through both the red and infrared channels. These mechanically-induced variances in the light's transmission and reception through the monitoring site can produce false arterial pulse waveforms that can mimic real waveforms. If the pulse oximeter cannot differentiate the motion-induced waveforms from true pulse waveforms, it will provide a value for O_2 saturation rather than indicate an error.

Figure 3.7 graphically displays data collected from the analog outputs of a pulse oximeter. The O_2 saturation signal (top panel) and arterial pulse waveform signal (middle panel) were collected with a personal computer and digitized at 50 Hz. Simultaneously, a three-lead ECG (bottom channel) was monitored and digitized at 50 Hz. The O_2 saturation signal is shown with a reduced resolution to illustrate signal stability. Arrows mark the corresponding times on each strip. These tracings emphasize that for each QRS complex seen and recorded on the ECG channel, a corresponding pulse waveform peak occurs

Figure 3.7— Arterial pulse waveforms, normal sinus rhythm, and stable oximetry reading.

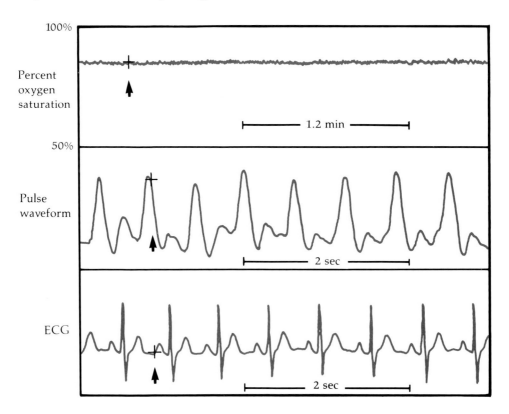

Figure 3.8— Arterial and secondary pulse waveforms, normal sinus rhythm, and unstable oximetry reading.

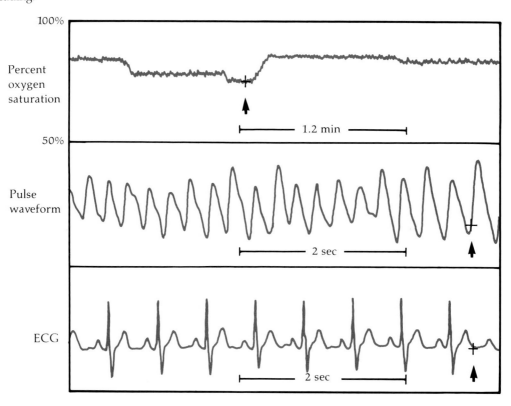

within approximately one-half second later. Since a peak-for-peak correlation between the pulse waveform and ECG channel exists, the value for O_2 saturation derived from the pulse waveform is representative of arterial blood.

Figure 3.8 presents signals collected from the same subject using the same collection and display paradigm as in Figure 3.7. Once again, the O_2 saturation signal is shown with a decreased resolution to illustrate signal stability, and arrows mark the corresponding points in time. This tracing highlights the effects of motion on the pulse waveform signal. Unlike Figure 3.7, in which clearly identified arterial pulse waveforms correspond with each QRS complex, this figure illustrates randomly-occurring pulse waveforms. The frequency and amplitude of these artifactually-induced waveforms are such that they elude the oximeter's filtering techniques. Therefore, the accuracy of the calculation of O_2 saturation is erroneous. For example, in this illustration, the pulse oximeter provides a value of 87% O_2 saturation, but the actual value of O_2 saturation is 96%.

One possible explanation of why pulse oximeters can calculate values of O_2 saturation from artifactually-induced changes in light intensity is that the artifactual pulse waveform may generate an AC signal larger in amplitude than the genuine, arterial pulse-modulated AC signal. Because of the artificially heightened pulse amplitude, the ratio of the red-to-infrared signals becomes almost entirely a function of a DC signal.[47] Because of their large amplitude, the voltage of the two signals is similar and their ratio to each other becomes one. The calibration curve that most pulse oximeters use to convert the ratio of absorbed red to infrared light defines a ratio of one as an O_2 saturation of about 84% to 88% (Figure 3.4). Unfortunately, since these values can be clinically reasonable, their authenticity can only be verified by an inspection of the pulse waveform's integrity from which they were calculated.

3.5.2   Cardiac Arrhythmias

Figure 3.9 illustrates O_2 saturation, pulse waveform, and electrocardiogram, using the same collection parameters as described in Figure 3.7. Occasional premature ventricular contractions (PVCs) are visible on the electrocardiogram. However, their presence did not sufficiently alter the morphology of the pulse waveform. Since the PVCs did not alter the pulse waveform's characteristics, the pulse oximeter accepted their validity and calculated values of O_2 saturation. If periodic cardiac arrhythmias would affect the morphology of the pulse waveform, the pulse oximeter's pulse waveform processing algorithm would process those waveforms as if they were artifact. Then the pulse oximeter's pulse waveform weighing, averaging, and rejection schemes should determine the acceptability of the incoming pulse waveform signals.

Cardiac arrhythmias that could be potentially detrimental to the pulse oximeter's ability to measure arterial O_2 saturation are those associated with sustained, decreased cardiac outputs. Sustained ventricular tachycardia, for example, is associated with sudden decreases in blood pressure due to inadequate cardiac filling time. This, in turn, could produce an insufficient pulse waveform that the pulse oximeter cannot measure.

3.5.3   Hypothermia

Patients in medical and surgical intensive care units who are hypothermic, whether induced by cooling mattresses intraoperatively or postoperatively, are subjected to peripheral vasoconstriction. Consequently, the vasoconstriction creates low pulse pressures with

Figure 3.9— Unstable pulse waveforms, ventricular extrasystoles, and stable oximeter readings.

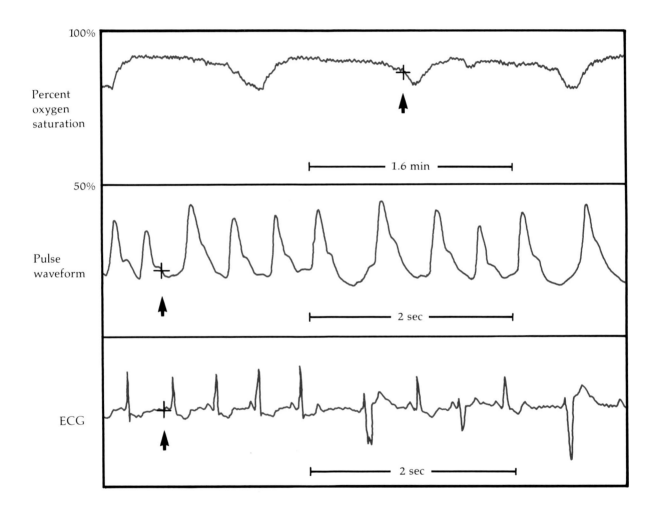

poor quality pulse waveforms. During these conditions, the amplitude of the pulse waveform may be so small that the pulse oximeter cannot accurately measure it. To compensate for the pulse-received waveform signal, the pulse oximeter raises the driving current of the LEDs as well as increases the gain of the photoreceiver to bring the measured amplitude of the pulse waveform into a workable range.[48] This increase in LED driving current and increased photoreceiver gain concomitantly increases the noise-to-signal ratio. As a result, the pulse oximeter becomes more susceptible to motion artifact and to other mechanisms that could create false values of O_2 saturation.

So, while the hypothermic condition itself has not been reported to cause oximeter error, the peripheral vasoconstriction associated with it may cause the pulse oximeter to become more susceptible to artifactually-induced signals.[49,50]

3.6 *Data Averaging and Artifact Rejection Schemes*

A small heart-beat-to-heart-beat variability in O_2 saturation does exist. This variability, observed in pulse oximeters that provide beat-by-beat displays of O_2 saturation, can be caused by the initial arterial pulse pressure compressing and emptying the venous bed. As the arterial pressure decreases, the venous bed opens and fills, behaving like an artery. Since the venous and arterial pulsations occur virtually simultaneously, a small amount of venous blood is detected by the oximeter and included in the calculation of O_2 saturation. The actual amount of blood remaining in the venous system may vary with heart rate, arterial blood pressure, or cardiac output, thereby creating pulse-to-pulse variations in measured O_2 saturation.

Displaying the pulse-to-pulse variations could prove somewhat distracting to the clinician. To help eliminate small variations in displayed O_2 saturation values, pulse oximeter algorithms use data smoothing schemes. Briefly, data smoothing averages the values of O_2 saturation over several heart beats to provide a single value. In turn, data smoothing can eliminate small pulse-to-pulse variations in the O_2 saturation signal. Also, during infrequent episodes of motion, any sporadic artifactual readings are averaged with the correct readings to help stabilize the signal and to prevent the display of erratic values of O_2 saturation.

The major problem with lengthy signal averaging routines is a delayed machine response time during acute changes in O_2 saturation. Also, imprecise displays of high and low O_2 saturation values during hypoxic events may occur since normative values immediately preceding and following the events are averaged in with the lower values. Therefore, a shorter signal or data-dependent filtering algorithm averaging time is more favorable since it helps minimize these errors.

To help counter the possibility of the pulse oximeter providing false values of O_2 saturation from artifactual pulse waveforms and to keep data averaging times to a minimum, the oximeter algorithm employs various artifact rejection schemes. Some pulse oximeters employ predefined templates of arterial pulse waveforms to which all incoming pulse waveforms are fitted. If the incoming pulse waveform does not fit the template, one of several events occurs depending upon the pulse oximeter being used. Some algorithms discard the pulse waveforms that do not fit within the template. If a string of unusable waveforms appear, the oximeter displays an error message. Other oximeter algorithms in the presence of unusable pulse waveforms freeze the last, correct O_2 saturation value. This value can be held in the display for several seconds or until usable waveforms reappear.

Another technique to filter out artifactual pulse waveforms employs weighted pulse waveform averaging schemes. This strategy applies a "weight" or a "measure" to the quality of the incoming pulse waveform. Values of O_2 saturation derived from pulse waveforms that have low weighted measure of their authenticity contribute minimally to the overall calculation of O_2 saturation. Pulse waveforms that have a large weighted measure for their authenticity contribute maximally to the calculation of O_2 saturation. Waveform weighing, when used in conjunction with pulse waveform templates, provides a fairly effective mechanism for separating artifact from the physiologic pulse waveform.

Most pulse oximeter manufacturers state that the accuracy of their machines are within 2% to 4% of actual arterial O_2 saturation values. As mentioned earlier, the value a pulse oximeter displays as O_2 saturation is termed "functional saturation". Functional saturation is the sum of the four hemoglobin species (both O_2-binding and nonoxygen-binding hemoglobins) present in the blood. The presence of dyshemoglobins accounts for a small portion of the red light absorbance which affects the oximeter's precision for its oxyhemoglobin measurement. Dyshemoglobins also account for 2% to 4% of the value that pulse oximeters display as "O_2 saturation". Therefore, the displayed value is 2% to 4% higher than the actual value of arterial O_2 saturation.

During profound hypoxemia, the error in pulse oximetric measurements of arterial O_2 saturation may be larger than the manufacturer's stated range. Many potential reasons explain the oximeter's inaccuracy during hypoxemia, but no one specific cause has been actually identified. Several plausible explanations why oximeters become less accurate at low levels of O_2 saturation have been proposed. One frequently mentioned reason involves the oximeter's initial calibration protocol.

As previously described, pulse oximeters are calibrated by attachment to a healthy human subject who breathes a hypoxic gas mixture. The limitation to this calibration technique is that most protocols only allow the subject to undergo desaturation to 75% arterial O_2 saturation. Some protocols do induce profound hypoxemia, but they are not commonly practiced during industrial pulse oximeter calibrating protocols. Therefore, since the pulse oximeter can only be calibrated with real human data down to a certain point, the lower end of the calibration curve must be extrapolated from the existing data. This extrapolation of data to a calibration curve can introduce measurement errors.

Another explanation of why pulse oximeters become less accurate at low O_2 saturation levels involves the light shunting theory as previously explained. To review, it is possible that, during hypoxemic conditions, a portion of the red light follows the path of least resistance around the periphery of the monitoring site instead of through the darkened blood. If any of the shunted light comes in contact with the unshunted light that has assumed AC characteristics, an overall increase in light intensity could occur. This could create an artifact in the red-to-infrared light ratios that would cause the pulse oximeter to produce erroneous values of O_2 saturation. While this scenario is theoretically feasible, it has yet to be scientifically validated.

Although these effects can potentially cause the pulse oximeter to overestimate actual arterial O_2 saturation during hypoxemic conditions, other previously described conditions can also produce pulse oximeter errors during hypoxemia. Of these, anemia, CO poisoning, and skin color (to some degree) are the most clinically relevant.

3.7   *Summary*

All currently available pulse oximeters use LEDs to transmit red and infrared light in the region of 660 nm and 940 nm, respectively. The light is transmitted through a vascular bed to a photoreceiver positioned opposite the LEDs. As the light passes through the vascular bed, its intensity is modulated by the filling and emptying of the arterioles, which affect both the red and the infrared lights. The red light is further modulated by the color of the hemoglobin, in that the darker the hemoglobin molecule, the more red light it absorbs. The photoreceiver positioned on the opposite of the LEDs measures the intensity of both the red and infrared light that passes through the vascular bed. From this, the ratio of red to infrared light is derived and used to determine arterial O_2 saturation.

When arterial O_2 is measured in vivo using pulse oximetry, the value produced is called SpO_2. In vitro measurements of arterial O_2 saturation, obtained by arterial puncture and co-oximetric analysis of the sample are known as SaO_2. Both pulse oximetry and co-oximetry measure O_2 bound to hemoglobin by light transmission and reception. The distinction is that co-oximetry uses multiple light wavelengths to produce separate measurements of both oxyhemoglobin and dyshemoglobins. Therefore, a value of SaO_2 produced by co-oximetry represents only O_2 bound to hemoglobin. On the other hand, pulse oximeters use only two light wavelengths, and therefore, cannot differentiate between oxyhemoglobin and dyshemoglobins. Consequently, they measure total hemoglobin saturation. Hence, SpO_2 is the sum of both the oxyhemoglobin and the dyshemoglobins levels.

Although pulse oximetry measurements are generally considered risk free, there have been reports of patients receiving burn injuries from pulse oximeter sensors.[51] Defective LEDs in the finger sensor have led to patients being burned on their fingertips during intraoperative pulse oximetry monitoring. Another source of patient burns is the connecting of one manufacturer's pulse oximeter sensor to another manufacturer's pulse oximeter. The sensor may connect without difficulty, but the pulse oximeter sends excessive electrical current to the LEDs causing them to overheat. To prevent these errors from occurring, some pulse oximeters send a signal through the sensor to identify its circuitry. If the sensor responds appropriately, and in a predetermined fashion, the pulse oximeter continues to operate. If the sensor does not respond appropriately, the pulse oximeter displays an error message and alarm.

While pulse oximeters may be adversely affected by specific environmental, physiological, or technical conditions, their convenience, minimal patient discomfort, and overall accuracy often outweigh these limitations. These factors encourage the future use of such devices in clinical settings. Therefore, clinicians who are familiar with the operating principles and the technical limitations of pulse oximetry are better equipped to use this technology to its fullest potential.[52]

Figure 4.1— The oxygen-hemoglobin dissociation
curve.

a   = normal arterial
v̄   = normal mixed venous
P_{50} = the partial pressure (27 mm Hg) at which
      Hb is 50% saturated.

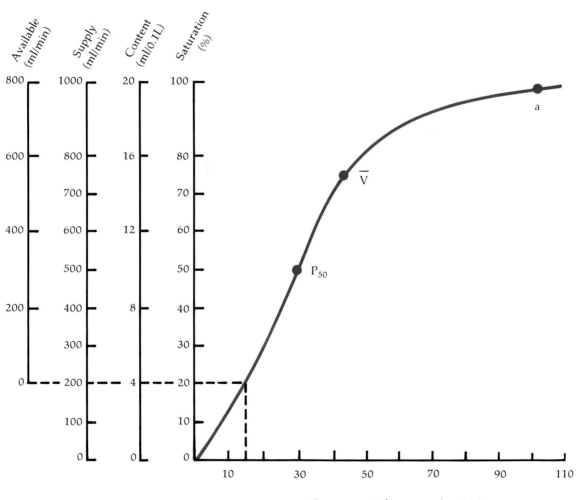

4.0 MIXED VENOUS OXYGEN SATURATION

Prior to the development of an accurate bedside monitor of the mixed venous oxygen ($S\bar{v}O_2$) saturation of hemoglobin, clinical management of cardiorespiratory problems relied on intermittent laboratory measurements of venous saturation. Early attempts at continuous $S\bar{v}O_2$ monitoring were unsuccessful for a variety of technical reasons. Clinical use of $S\bar{v}O_2$ has increased dramatically following the development of an accurate bedside monitor. In this chapter the development, basic physiology, pathophysiology and clinical applications of $S\bar{v}O_2$ are reviewed.

4.1 General Principles and History

4.1.1 Relation to the Fick Principle

The Fick principle states that cardiac output (CO) can be determined from knowing the oxygen consumed (VO_2) and the difference in O_2 content of blood leaving and returning to the lungs:

$$CO = \frac{VO_2}{C_aO_2 - C_{\bar{v}}O} \qquad \text{Equation 4.1}$$

where
C_aO_2 = O_2 content of arterial blood
$C_{\bar{v}}O_2$ = O_2 content of mixed venous blood

Oxygen content in blood (CO_2) is determined by the sum of: 1) The hemoglobin concentration multiplied by 1.39 (the milliliters O_2 per gram of hemoglobin), multiplied by the percent of hemoglobin that is saturated, and 2) its solubilized portion in plasma of 0.003 milliliters per mm Hg O_2 tension in blood (PO_2).

This is expressed as:

$$CO_2 = (1.39)(Hb)(SaO_2) + (0.003)(PO_2) \qquad \text{Equation 4.2}$$

where
SaO_2* = percent O_2 saturation of arterial Hb (x.01)

*The value for SpO_2 (as obtained from pulse oximetry) can be substituted in equations denoting arterial O_2 saturation. The term SaO_2 is used throughout this text for clarity.

Because of the small relative contribution of the plasma-soluble fraction at usual partial pressures of O_2, the equation for the clinically significant O_2 content of blood can be simplified to:

$$CO_2 = (1.39)(Hb)(SaO_2) \qquad \text{Equation 4.3}$$

Rearrangement of the Fick equation can then yield calculation of O_2 consumption by:

Figure 4.2— Oxygen extraction from various organs.

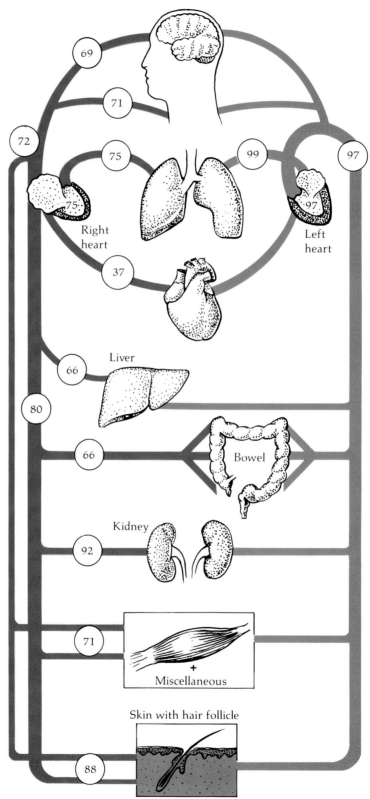

$$V_{O_2} = (CO)[C_{(a-v)}O_2]$$ **Equation 4.4**

where $C_{(a-v)}O_2 = $ arterial-venous difference in C_{O_2}

And, by substitution for C_{O_2}:

$$V_{O_2} = (CO)(1.39)(Hb)(SaO_2 - S\bar{v}O_2)$$ **Equation 4.5**

It is then necessary only to measure $S\bar{v}O_2$ in calculating systemic O_2 consumption. Knowing the SaO_2 by noninvasive pulse oximetry and the cardiac output, O_2 delivery can be quantified.

As noted above, these calculations are valid assuming normal O_2 tensions and hemoglobin concentrations. Because hemoglobin saturation will not change at P_aO_2s in excess of 150 mm Hg (Figure 4.1), SaO_2 measurement is an insensitive indicator of C_aO_2 changes in those ranges. For the anemic patient with a high P_aO_2, the relative contribution of the plasma-soluble O_2 fraction to the overall C_aO_2 can become significant, and should be considered.

4.1.2 Site of S$\bar{v}$O$_2$ Measurement

The $S\bar{v}O_2$ reflects the balance between O_2 delivery and O_2 consumption in the body as a whole. Sampling of true mixed venous blood can therefore only be obtained from the pulmonary artery, since O_2 extraction varies from different regions and organ systems and mixing is therefore incomplete proximal to this site (Figure 4.2).

4.1.3 Determinants of Oxygen Delivery

Oxygen delivery is calculated by multiplying the C_aO_2 by the cardiac output. The C_aO_2 is most sensitive to the hemoglobin concentration in blood and the saturation of hemoglobin with O_2. The influence of hemoglobin concentration on C_aO_2 is proportional and occurs in a linear fashion, although hemoglobin concentrations above 15 gm/dl increase blood viscosity to the point of compromising local tissue perfusion and O_2 delivery.[53] The shape of the oxyhemoglobin dissociation curve (Figure 4.1) reflects the fact that saturation of hemoglobin remains virtually unchanged when the O_2 tension is 150 mm Hg or greater, although saturation drops dramatically below an O_2 tension in the area of 60 mm Hg.

Cardiac output is the flow of blood delivered to the peripheral circulation, commonly measured in liters per minute (LPM), and can be effected by changes in volume loading (preload), changes in resistance to flow (afterload), changes in myocardial contractility, and heart rate.

4.1.4 Determinants of Oxygen Demand

Oxygen demand is the amount of O_2 required by the body's tissues in a given time. Oxygen consumption, to meet this demand, again can be determined by the Fick equation, or measured directly with calorimetry. Oxygen demand in the normal resting adult is 5 ml O_2 from every 100 ml of blood flow.[54] Assuming a C_aO_2 of 20 dl/ml blood at 100% hemoglobin saturation, an $S\bar{v}O_2$ of 75% can be predicted at steady state. A baseline O_2 consumption can be calculated by factoring in the cardiac output (using Equation 4.4):

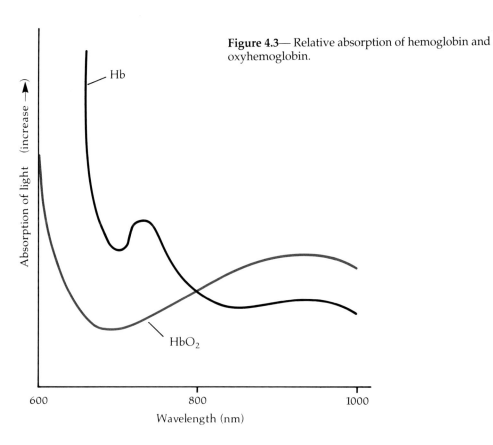

Figure 4.3— Relative absorption of hemoglobin and oxyhemoglobin.

Figure 4.4— Relative reflection of hemoglobin and oxyhemoglobin.

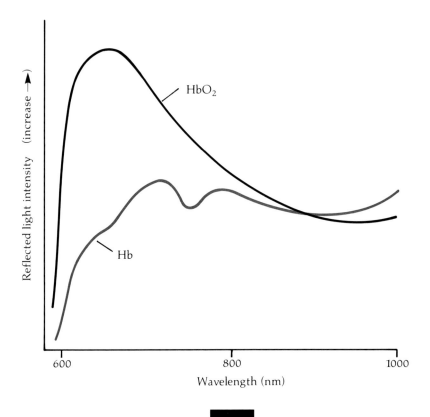

$$VO_2 = (C_aO_2 - C_vO_2) \times CO \qquad \text{Equation 4.6}$$

where

$$CO = 5.0 \text{ LPM}$$

$$VO_2 = (20 \text{ dl } O_2/\text{ml} - 15 \text{ dl } O_2/\text{ml})(5 \text{ LPM})(10 \text{ dl}/\text{l})$$

$$VO_2 = 250 \text{ ml/min.}$$

Oxygen demand can change through a variety of factors as discussed below.

4.1.5 Historical Development of Saturation Monitoring

In 1935, Kramer first demonstrated a method of measuring O_2 saturation in flowing blood on a continuous basis.[55] He originally did this by galvanometrically measuring the blood's absorption of an incandescent light shone through a red filter with a photocell. Later, in 1939, Matthes and Gross described a combined red and infrared O_2 saturation meter that measured transmittance through the ear. Millikan refined this concept to a more practical design in the early 1940s and first coined the term "oximeter".[56,57] Modern oximeters continue to apply these concepts, measuring the transmission and absorbance of red and infrared light sources in blood and comparing the results with known values for oxyhemoglobin and reduced hemoglobin (Figure 4.3).

Brinkman and Zijlstra first described the measurement of O_2 saturation by reflected light in 1949.[58] Their original method used reflected red light as measured from the forehead. Their theories of reflection oximetry paved the way for the fiberoptic catheters (Figure 4.4).

Polanyi, working with the American Optical Company, developed a reflection-oximeter using optical fibers during the late 1950s. Working with Cournand, clinical application of his designs were implemented using a cardiac catheter in 1962.[59,60] These early catheters were limited in their usefulness, however, by the fragility of their fibers, the overall size of the catheters, and their inability to provide consistent measurements in the face of changing hemoglobin concentrations.

4.1.6 Current Technological Features and Applications

Improvements in fiberoptics and the development of pulmonary artery catheters have allowed the integration of these technologies with reflection spectrophotometry, making bedside $S\bar{v}O_2$ monitoring possible (Figure 4.5). The most accurate commercially-available system uses three wavelengths of light, which is superior to two-wavelength systems for measuring abrupt changes in $S\bar{v}O_2$ of patients with stable hemoglobin concentrations (Figure 4.6).[61,62]

Other technological improvements include a processing algorithm using continuous ratios to reduce vessel wall artifact and LEDs for the narrow-band source. These developments enable the system to produce accurate measurements of continuous $S\bar{v}O_2$ over a wide range of hemoglobin concentrations. Such advances have improved the accuracy and usefulness of $S\bar{v}O_2$.

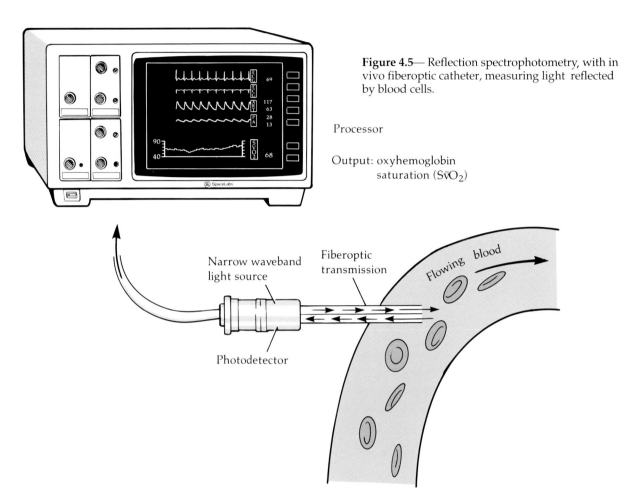

Figure 4.5— Reflection spectrophotometry, with in vivo fiberoptic catheter, measuring light reflected by blood cells.

Processor

Output: oxyhemoglobin
saturation ($S\bar{v}O_2$)

Narrow waveband light source

Fiberoptic transmission

Flowing blood

Photodetector

Figure 4.6 — The catheter used with the Oximetrix optical oximetry system.

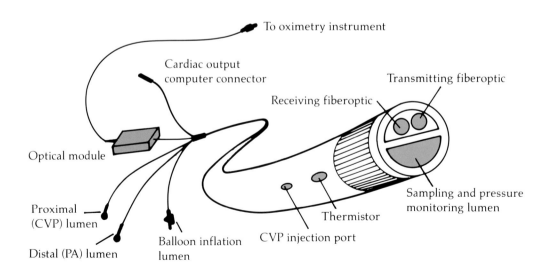

Fiberoptic catheter

To oximetry instrument

Cardiac output computer connector

Transmitting fiberoptic

Receiving fiberoptic

Optical module

Proximal (CVP) lumen

Distal (PA) lumen

Balloon inflation lumen

CVP injection port

Thermistor

Sampling and pressure monitoring lumen

4.2   *Physiologic Conditions Monitored by S$\bar{v}$O$_2$*

S$\bar{v}$O$_2$ provides an indication of the O$_2$ remaining in mixed venous blood following use by the tissues, thus reflecting the balance between O$_2$ delivery and consumption. The residual amount of O$_2$ in venous blood depends not only on the amount of O$_2$ consumed in the tissues, but is also dependent upon the variables of arterial saturation, hemoglobin concentration, and cardiac output. The amount of actual O$_2$ consumption by the tissues is also a dynamic process usually independent of these factors. As such, S$\bar{v}$O$_2$ is a sensitive but nonspecific indicator of the relationship between delivery and consumption.

4.2.1   Adequacy of Oxygen Delivery

The variables of O$_2$ delivery (SaO$_2$, hemoglobin concentration, and cardiac output) can be considered independent. However, with knowledge of two out of three variables it is possible to make reasonably accurate estimates of the adequacy of the third parameter.

When hemoglobin concentration, SaO$_2$, and O$_2$ consumption are considered constant, changes in S$\bar{v}$O$_2$ are likely to result from a change in cardiac output. Clinically, in such situations the alterations in O$_2$ consumption occur either slowly or in response to some sudden, but obvious, change in demand. Likewise, variations in hemoglobin concentration occur slowly even in a patient who is acutely bleeding, due to the slow refilling of the plasma component. Therefore, when the SaO$_2$ is known and constant, the C$_{(a-v)}$O$_2$ as measured knowing the S$\bar{v}$O$_2$ will tell whether cardiac output is adequate in meeting O$_2$ consumption based on the Fick principle (Equation 4.5).

An unchanging S$\bar{v}$O$_2$ trend usually indicates a stable relationship between the components of O$_2$ delivery and consumption. A changing trend should alert the clinician to reexamine the patient to detect any changes that might require therapy.

4.2.2   Increased Oxygen Demand

Many clinical conditions can result in increased O$_2$ demand. One simple example is the exercising athlete who requires increased O$_2$ for working skeletal musculature. While the athlete can compensate for increased demand through large increases in cardiac output, he or she may also demonstrate a marked increase in C$_{(a-v)}$O$_2$ (measured as a decrease in S$\bar{v}$O$_2$), reflecting increased O$_2$ consumption. This same principle holds in pathologic states of increased O$_2$ demand, and changes in C$_{(a-v)}$O$_2$ are even more dramatic in those patients with a compromised ability to increase their cardiac output.

4.2.3   Inadequate Oxygen Consumption

While O$_2$ demand represents the overall O$_2$ requirements of the body, O$_2$ consumption defines the utilization of delivered O$_2$ by the body as a whole. S$\bar{v}$O$_2$ does not directly measure the balance between O$_2$ demand and consumption, but it can reflect the ability of compensatory adjustments to meet that changing demand.

When the body is unable to adequately obtain O$_2$ to meet demand, the result is anaerobic metabolism, which is measured by the presence of lactic acidosis. Anaerobic metabolism represents either inadequate O$_2$ delivery or an inability of the tissues to extract

Figure 4.7— Oxygen-hemoglobin dissociation curve as affected by changes in pH, Pco_2, and temperature.

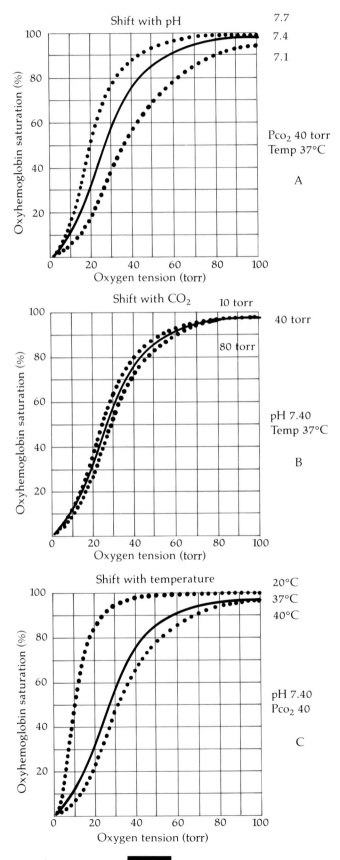

O_2. Excluding the latter cause, continuous $S\bar{v}O_2$ monitoring may be used to determine the presence of ongoing anaerobic metabolism and the adequacy of O_2 consumption in lactic acidosis.[63]

Body temperature, pH, $P_{C}O_2$, and 2, 3-diphosphoglycerate affect the binding of O_2 to hemoglobin and thus can change O_2 consumption (Figure 4.7). The resulting change in O_2 consumption is seen as a change in $S\bar{v}O_2$.

4.3 *Clinical Applications*

The normal $S\bar{v}O_2$ in the resting adult is 75%, although the acceptable range may vary from 60% to 80%. The threshold signaling induction of anaerobic metabolism is approximately 50%.[64]

4.3.1 Oxygen Delivery

The determinants of O_2 delivery, cardiac output, SaO_2, and hemoglobin concentration are all represented to varying degrees in a number of pathologic states. These measures, in turn, are reflected by changes in $S\bar{v}O_2$.

The relationship between cardiac output and $S\bar{v}O_2$, based on the Fick principle, is not linear (Figure 4.8). In patients with low cardiac output states, small changes in output can result in quite large changes of the $C_{(a-v)}O_2$. Taking this into consideration, alterations in cardiac output and the resultant effects on the O_2 delivery/consumption balance can be assessed and can guide therapy towards changing the cardiac output. Changes in cardiac output indicated by $S\bar{v}O_2$ may be noticeable prior to changes in heart rate, mean arterial pressure (MAP), or pulmonary artery occlusion pressure (PAOP).[65]

SaO_2 values can be altered as a result of changes in minute ventilation, diffusion capacity within the lungs, fractional inspired oxygen concentration (FiO_2), or positive end-expiratory pressure (PEEP). Changes in SaO_2 can also be caused by intrapulmonary shunting or ventilation-perfusion inequalities.

The relationship between hemoglobin concentration and $S\bar{v}O_2$ is linear. Low $S\bar{v}O_2$ values may indicate the need for a blood transfusion because of inadequate O_2 delivery.[66]

4.3.2 Oxygen Consumption

Changes in $S\bar{v}O_2$ reflect a variety of pathologic states, either from disease or from iatrogenic manipulations. Increases in O_2 consumption may result from exercise, agitation or pain, shivering, hypermetabolism from thyroid dysfunction or malignant hyperthermia, infectious diseases, hypersensitivity reactions, and rewarming after cardiopulmonary bypass. Decreases in O_2 consumption may result from hypothermia, or from general anesthesia through cutaneous vasodilation, decreased muscle tone, and heat generation.

The assessment of O_2 consumption in the critical care setting is extremely important in determining the patient's response to shock. Maintenance of normal or supranormal O_2 consumption has been correlated with improved outcome in these patients.[67] In addition, O_2 consumption may decrease early on in these states prior to the manifestation of other hemodynamic changes.[68]

Figure 4.8—Calculated relationship between cardiac index (CI) and $S\bar{v}O_2$ at constant Vo_2 and C_aO_2

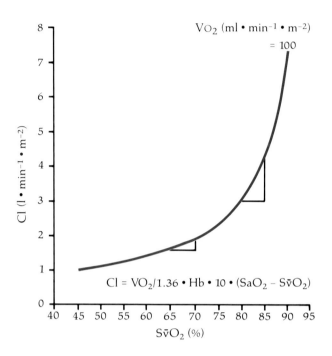

VO_2 (ml • min^{-1} • m^{-2}) = 100

CI (l • min^{-1} • m^{-2})

$CI = VO_2/1.36 • Hb • 10 • (SaO_2 − S\bar{v}O_2)$

$S\bar{v}O_2$ (%)

Figure 4.9—Iso-shunt diagram. Bands represent various values of Hb concentration.

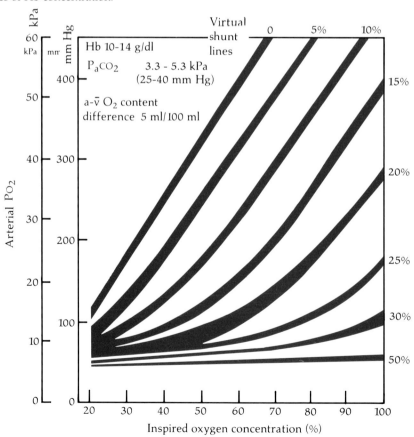

Virtual shunt lines

Hb 10-14 g/dl
P_aCO_2 3.3 - 5.3 kPa
          (25-40 mm Hg)

a-$\bar{v}$ O_2 content
difference 5 ml/100 ml

Arterial PO_2

Inspired oxygen concentration (%)

4.3.3   Pulmonary Blood Flow

When cardiac output decreases or O_2 consumption increases, and the intrapulmonary shunt fraction ($\dot{Q}sp/\dot{Q}t$) remains constant, tissues must extract more O_2 per unit volume of blood and, therefore decrease $S\bar{v}O_2$. Progressive increases in $\dot{Q}sp/\dot{Q}t$ present more desaturated venous blood to the arterial side, decreasing C_aO_2, and potentially resulting in a vicious cycle. Determination of $\dot{Q}sp/\dot{Q}t$ can be derived from $S\bar{v}O_2$ if the oxygenation of end-pulmonary capillary blood (c´ flow) is known by:

$$\dot{Q}sp/\dot{Q}t \;=\; \frac{Sc´O_2 - SaO_2}{Sc´O_2 - S\bar{v}O_2}$$

Equation 4.7

where $\qquad\qquad Sc´O_2 \;=\; O_2$ saturation of c´ flow
(assuming $Pc´O_2 \;=\;$ alveolar PO_2).

At shunts approaching 50%, O_2 delivery no longer responds to increasing FiO_2, (Figure 4.9) and therapy must be directed at decreasing the shunt.[69]

4.3.4   Optimal Mechanical Ventilation

Because $S\bar{v}O_2$ is a reliable indicator in most tissue oxygenation states, its monitoring helps in assessing the effectiveness of various manipulations upon patients who are mechanically ventilated. The usefulness of $S\bar{v}O_2$ has been well-documented for determining optimal levels of PEEP.[70,71] In patients for whom PEEP increases arterial hemoglobin saturation and PO_2, the $S\bar{v}O_2$ usually improves. Excessive PEEP decreases cardiac output and $S\bar{v}O_2$. The optimal level of PEEP is the one resulting in the best $S\bar{v}O_2$.

4.3.5   Pulmonary Artery Catheter Position

Use of $S\bar{v}O_2$ monitoring allows confirmation of true wedge by the pulmonary artery catheter through its ability to detect the increase in O_2 saturation that occurs when measuring pulmonary capillary blood flow. Further confirmation can, of course, be obtained by withdrawing capillary wedge blood from the catheter tip. Perhaps more important is the ability to detect distal catheter migration, a frequent occurrence with potentially disastrous consequences.[72,73] Because the fiberoptic catheter continuously reads the intensity of the light being reflected, the changes associated with migration into a wedge can be identified by the computer unit; preset alarms can warn of the event.

4.3.6   Cost-Effectiveness in the Critical Care Setting

One of the more useful aspects of $S\bar{v}O_2$ monitoring is its function as a trend monitor. This characteristic helps the clinician determine when various patient profiling, such as arterial blood gas analysis, determination of hemoglobin concentration, or cardiac output measurement, is indicated. Furthermore, $S\bar{v}O_2$ monitoring allows the clinician to reduce the number of these routine measurements when the patient is stable. It is also a potential method for analyzing the effects of various changes in treatment without the delay and cost of other tests. The proper use of this continuous monitoring technology could eliminate the waste of resources that are often "protocol"-based.[74] However, it is unclear at which point in a patient's care the use of this particular monitoring becomes economically favorable.[75]

4.4 *Limitations of S$\bar{v}$O$_2$ Monitoring*

4.4.1 Nonspecificity

S$\bar{v}$O$_2$ monitoring does not determine the source of imbalances between O$_2$ delivery and consumption, but only reflects the total O$_2$ reserve of the entire body. Oxygen consumption within a given organ system can be maintained in the face of limited O$_2$ delivery through increased extraction.[76] Conversely, severe individual organ system O$_2$ imbalance can occur with an apparently normal S$\bar{v}$O$_2$.

4.4.2 Disease States

One of the pathologic states best known to confound the reliability of S$\bar{v}$O$_2$ monitoring is that of sepsis. Septic patients have been described as having a pathologic dependence of O$_2$ consumption upon O$_2$ delivery.[77] This dependency may represent distributive inadequacies of tissue oxygenation despite supranormal O$_2$ delivery.[77] The same dependency has been seen in patients with adult respiratory distress syndrome, congestive heart failure, and hepatic failure, and after cardiopulmonary bypass. Other evidence, using independent measurements of O$_2$ delivery and consumption in septic patients with stable hemodynamics, indicates that these patients fail to demonstrate this pathologic O$_2$ supply dependency.[78] Still, caution must be advised in evaluating S$\bar{v}$O$_2$ measurements from septic patients since normal or even high S$\bar{v}$O$_2$ values can coexist with actual tissue hypoxia.[79]

Acute myocardial infarction appears to limit the reliability of S$\bar{v}$O$_2$ measurements in predicting changes in cardiac output.[80] This breakdown in reliability has been associated with an unstable rate of O$_2$ consumption at the tissue level. It has been recommended that a relationship between measured cardiac output and S$\bar{v}$O$_2$ be established for unstable patients prior to use of S$\bar{v}$O$_2$ as a monitoring parameter.[81,82]

Patients with chronically low cardiac output states and chronic obstructive pulmonary disease appear to function at baseline levels despite subnormal S$\bar{v}$O$_2$.[83,84] These cases represent the adaptability of the various compensatory mechanisms to maintain O$_2$ consumption despite compromised delivery. Because the reserves of these patients are already compromised or exhausted, their susceptability to any further insult must be kept in mind. On the other hand, efforts to always treat the S$\bar{v}$O$_2$ value by itself can prove fruitless and ill-advised; the number is not the disease.

Diseases that affect O$_2$ loading and release from hemoglobin, such as hemoglobinopathies and various acid-base disturbances, can also alter S$\bar{v}$O$_2$ reliability. However, acute changes in S$\bar{v}$O$_2$ in such patients still indicate alterations in the DO$_2$-VO$_2$ balance and overall tissue oxygenation.

4.5 *New Technologies*

4.5.1 Additional Wavelength Analysis

While the development of a three-wavelength-measuring oximeter has improved the accuracy of $S\bar{v}O_2$ monitoring over a wider range of hemoglobin concentrations, methemoglobinemia and other dyshemoglobinemias produce significant errors in current $S\bar{v}O_2$ measurements.[85]

SaO$_2$ calculations from the Lambert-Beer law require separate wavelengths and equations for each type of hemoglobin measured (for example, four separate wavelengths to measure oxyhemoglobin, reduced hemoglobin, methemoglobin, and carboxyhemoglobin). However, this technology is not yet available for continuous in vivo bedside monitoring.

4.5.2 Dual Oximetry

One technology that is becoming more available is dual oximetry.[86] This method measures SaO$_2$ and S$\bar{v}$O$_2$ in real-time. It further integrates the data to allow calculation of the ventilation-perfusion index, estimation of $\dot{Q}sp/\dot{Q}t$, and analysis of O$_2$ extraction, and utilization.

5.0 IMPEDANCE PNEUMOGRAPHY

The first clinical use of thoracic impedance to monitor respiratory effort occurred in the 1960s with the recognition of prolonged apnea as a frequent problem for preterm infants.[87] The continuous recording of breathing patterns to document the behavior of infants at all ages was introduced in the 1970s.[88] The possibility to track all the physiologic variations created as breathing is generated by the complex interaction of the chest and abdomen in different body positions and sleep states.[89] The capacity to document the volume of ventilation is increasingly seen as a clinical need for patients of all ages, beyond the capacity of devices that create a simple estimate of breathing frequency. This has been apparent as breathing is monitored in adult patients after depo-narcotic anesthesia, and after withdrawing artificial ventilatory support in patients of all ages.[90]

While a number of respiratory-effort transducers have been devised (Table 5.1) practical considerations in the clinical environment initially has resulted in widespread use of thoracic impedance, principally because electrodes for electrocardiography are already in place. Thoracic impedance is usually detected between two ECG electrodes by passing a constant high frequency (20 to 100 kHz), low amperage current (<100 microamps) in a modified Einthoven Lead I or II position.[88] Despite its limitations, this somewhat imprecise technology has achieved wide clinical acceptance in equipment used to monitor patients in North America.[91]

Figure 5.1— Respitatory impedance as a vector.

Thoracic respiratory impedance change variables

Symbol	Name	Comment
ΔZ	Respiratory impedance change	Vector
$\lvert \Delta Z \rvert$	Magnitude of impedance change	Scalar
$\Delta \lvert Z \rvert$	Change of magnitude of impedance	Scalar
$\Delta \theta$	Phase angle change	Scalar
ΔR	Resistive or real part change	Scalar
ΔX_c	Capacitive or imaginary part change	Scalar

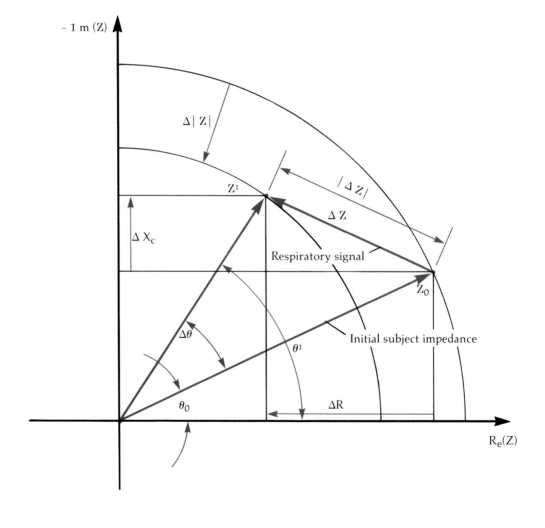

Table 5.1—Different types of respiratory effort transducers.

Respiration Effort Transducers	Air Flow Transducers
Thoracic impedance	Pneumotachometer
Pneumatic tube	Hot wire anemometer
Magnetometers	Ultrasound
Inductive belt	CO_2 [differential (qualitative), and tidal CO_2]
Mercury in rubber gauge	Thermistor
Electrolyte in rubber gauge	
Pressure capsule	
Mattresses (pneumatic, capacitance, electric)	

Thoracic impedance monitors have limitations in accurately depicting tidal volume, either as the actual volume ventilated effectively or the "volume" of respiratory effort generated against obstruction or restriction of air movement.[92] Most currently employed respiratory effort monitors focus on, at most, one of the two interacting body compartments that create the tidal volume.[93] Because the principle path of the current generating the impedance signal is superficial, it has been difficult to obtain an accurate indication of breathing volume even in those monitors using a lead II position.[94] In addition, ECG electrodes are most often in the position for optimal depiction of the QRS voltage while breathing patterns play a secondary role in virtually all adult CCUs and ICUs.

Many neonatal intensive care units in Europe use separate, disposable abdominal transducers of respiration in addition to ECG electrodes.[95] In both North America and Europe, most sleep physiology, pulmonary and neurodiagnostic centers have used transducers around both the thoracic and abdominal compartments.[96] This section describes in detail the theoretical and practical aspects of thoracic impedance measurement simply because of its current widespread use in bedside clinical monitors.

5.1 *Impedance*

5.1.1 **Methodology**

Impedance can be described (Figure 5.1) as a vector composed of capacitance and resistance.[97] The output of a bridge circuit is proportional to the change in impedance when the impedance (and phase angle) of resistance and capacitance are are equivalent to those of the patients impedance. With the constant current circuit, the output voltage is linearly proportional to patients impedance and the change in impedance. In an in-vitro cell of simple exact geometry, the impedance of an homogenous aqueous solution detected by a

Figure 5.2— Relationship of elastic tubing and frequency.

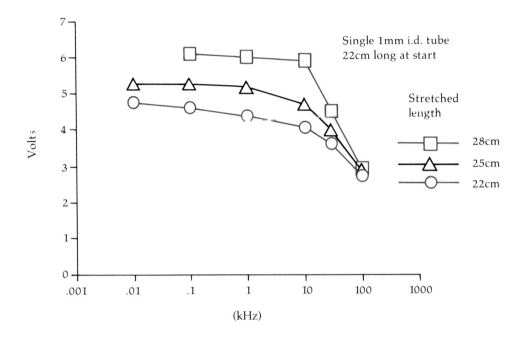

Single 1mm i.d. tube
22cm long at start

Stretched
length

28cm
25cm
22cm

Figure 5.3— Transducer made of a pair of tubes in parallel.

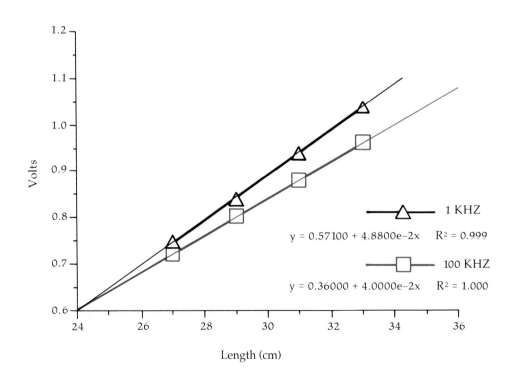

1 KHZ

y = 0.57100 + 4.8800e-2x   R² = 0.999

100 KHZ

y = 0.36000 + 4.0000e-2x   R² = 1.000

tetrapolar circuit gives a very accurate indication of the distance between the sampling electrodes at a frequency of 5000 Hz. Variations in salt concentration produce altered resistivity, but do not affect the measurement of the cell constant, especially in the ranges that commonly occur clinically. The major limitations in applying this precise measurement in the body are the effects of a complex geometry and the presence of multiple, non-homogenous current pathways.[98]

5.1.2 Elastic Transducer

If a long thin column of electrolyte is captured in an elastic tubing the relationship to frequency variations is more complex (Figure 5.2). This illustration shows the marked attenuation in signal dimension that occurs with increased frequency in the long narrow pathway within an elastic transducer filled with a highly conductive aqueous gel. The transducer was in series with a megohm resistor and a square wave signal of 20 volts p-p was used to produce the voltages recorded. Notice the variations in signal amplitude as the transducer is stretched from 22 cm to 28 cm in length at 1.0 kHz and 100 kHz.

Interestingly, at a fixed frequency with the correct range of tubing length and diameter, the impedance will vary linearly as the tubing length (cell distance) is increased. This has been demonstrated in a new form of transducer that gives a linear change in impedance when stretched from 1% to over 50% of its original linear dimension.[99] In Figure 5.3 the impedance of a pair of transducers in parallel shows a linear response to stretch and no interference generated by the second pathway in producing an exact relationship with stretch. The circumference change needed to characterize the full vital capacity (largest tidal volume, or 8 to 9 liters) will create no more than a 9-cm stretch on such a transducer. This transducer would allow the absolute dimension of the chest or abdomen to be monitored without a need to AC-couple the signal. This contained and more controlled use of impedance may allow for the development of respiration sensors that are quantitative, calibrated, non-toxic, non-restrictive, and inexpensive. Only a transducing technique with significant advantages in all five areas will displace the use of thoracic impedance measurements, despite the limitations in the technique.

5.1.3 Thoracic Tissue

Unfortunately, when the current is transmitted directly through the extremely complex and changing pathways in the human chest, the quantitative aspects of the signal are often lost. There is theoretical and experimental evidence to suggest that much of the usual variation of 0.1 to 5 Ohms that represents the signal of breathing effort on a base signal of 500 to 1000 Ohms is actually due to chest wall distortion rather than the direct measurement of lung expansion.[100] This is often due to uncontrollable physiologic variation in the tissue pathways that increase or decrease the signal amplitude independently of the amount of air being moved in and out of the lungs.[101] Figure 5.4 indicates that a large portion of the current created when thoracic impedance is measured actually travels in the chest wall.

5.1.3.1 Basal Impedance

The commonly seen base impedance using standard pediatric or adult ECG electrodes is approximately 500 Ohms for patients of all body sizes.[102] This observation leads to the

Figure 5.4— Current paths around and through the thoracic.

Base	Impedance	Variation
Artificial ventilation	500Ω	1Ω
Saline into trachea	425Ω	1Ω
Massage chest	425-430Ω	5Ω
Withdraw saline	490Ω	1Ω
Open chest and remove heart & lungs	570Ω	—

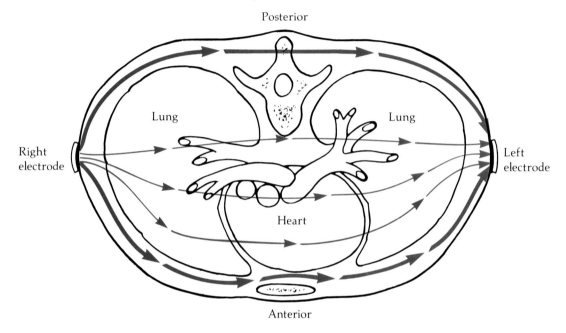

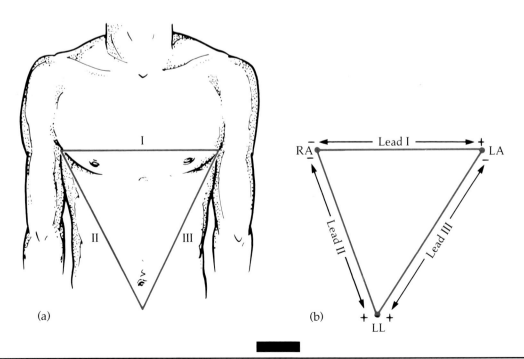

conclusion that chest wall thickness is appropriately increased as the transthoracic diameter increases with body size. If the measurement were dependent simply on the shortest direct physical path across the chest the same base impedance would not be observed in patients of widely different body sizes. This base impedance is also very dependent on the circuit-skin interface and increases markedly as the electrode contacts become "dried out". The capacitative component of the signal in human tissue has only been documented in a few articles.[103]

5.1.3.2 Bipolar Electrode

Figure 5.5 depicts a common bipolar electrode attachment for measuring thoracic impedance. The initial base impedance is about 500 Ohms through standard ECG electrodes in a modified lead I configuration. The signal is generated by a constant-current source at a frequency of 20,000 to 100,000 Hz with many monitors using values near 30,000 Hz. Multiple sites for attachment have been investigated, and the best correlation to tidal volume for seated adults occurred with an anterior-to-posterior attachment rather than the modified lead I or II usually used.[104] Not only is that anterior-posterior placement a non-standard ECG lead attachment; it is also far less comfortable for supine adult patients, so it is seldom employed clinically. It is also possible that using any pair of thoracic sites for a horizontal subject would not produce the same degree of correlation with the tidal volume that was seen in seated adults (Section 5.2).

5.1.3.3 Tetrapolar Electrode

Tetrapolar systems have been designed to reduce the complex effects from electrochemical reaction within the tissues at the electrode-skin interface by separating the activation and detection sites.[105] While a number of experimental approaches have been described, so far the advantages necessary to guarantee clinical acceptance of this more expensive and complex attachment have not been apparent. The signal detection problems with these systems are complicated by a significant reduction in signal strength.[106]

5.1.4 Other Uses of Impedance

The increase and decrease of blood in the path generating the thoracic impedance signal will produce a change with each heart beat.[107] Using alternative electrodes and a cephalad-to-caudad placement, some clinical researchers have achieved a degree of success in analyzing this pulse dimension and calculating a relationship with cardiac output.[108] Body composition and imaging have been attempted by impedance analysis. This is achieved without electrode contact by analyzing the pattern of disturbance in an electromagnetic field or saline bath.[109] The transmission of signals across the lower extremities has successfully been used to estimate peripheral limb blood flow and blood vessel variations.[110] While these techniques have been of interest for research, no routine volumetric clinical use of the signals has been employed except for peripheral blood flow. Whatever potential value may exist for the cardiologist, the cardiovascular component of the impedance signal is an artifact in a respiration circuit and a major source of error.[111]

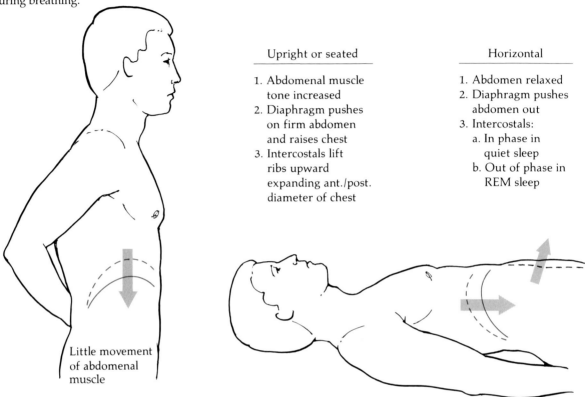

Figure 5.6— Effects of body position on muscles during breathing.

Upright or seated

1. Abdomenal muscle tone increased
2. Diaphragm pushes on firm abdomen and raises chest
3. Intercostals lift ribs upward expanding ant./post. diameter of chest

Horizontal

1. Abdomen relaxed
2. Diaphragm pushes abdomen out
3. Intercostals:
    a. In phase in quiet sleep
    b. Out of phase in REM sleep

Little movement of abdomenal muscle

Figure 5.7— The effect of sleep on movement of the chest and abdomen.

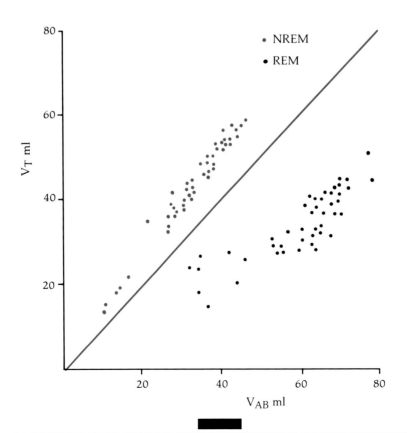

5.2 *Physiology of Breathing in Relation to Impedance Pneumography*

As described in Section 1.0, several midbrain and medullary centers produce the neural output to stimulate breathing activity.[112] These impulses travel over the appropriate cranial, phrenic, intercostal, and vertebral nerves to affect the tone of muscles that stabilize the airways and alter the compliance of the chest and abdomen.[113,114] These centers also signal the intermittent contractions that cause the expansion of either, or both, of these muscle-encased body compartments in order to expand the lungs.[115] The condition and response of this wide range of muscle groups will determine the adequacy of breathing. The most basic coordination of this activity is often not present for weeks after preterm birth.[116] The more stable breathing reflexes of term infants gradually develop and change toward a normal adult pattern of response.[117]

The three major muscles of breathing effort are: the diaphragm, the intercostals, and the anterior abdominal wall. The diaphragm is the principle muscle used in quiet ventilation.[118] The body compartments expanding as the diaphragm contracts will be altered by body position as in Figure 5.6. The fraction of the tidal volume causing expansion of the chest is large (40% to 60%) when the adults studied were seated, and became small (10% to 30%) compared to a much larger abdominal expansion that occurs when they are in a horizontal position.[118]

Movement of the chest and abdomen with inspiration occurs in three patterns: 1. When the subject is erect or seated, the anterior abdominal wall is firm and expansion is principally at the chest. 2. As the abdominal tone relaxes during horizontal breathing when awake or in quiet sleep, inspiration occurs at both the chest and abdomen, but principally the abdomen. 3. In horizontal breathing in active or REM sleep, or even more completely with airway obstruction, the abdomen generates much more change in volume than indicated by the tidal volume of gas moved.[119]

In the third pattern, the volume of gas displacement is reduced by a negative, passive inward movement of the chest wall, reducing the amount of chest volume available for lung expansion as the diaphragm contracts on inspiration. This occurs when the intercostal muscle tone supporting the chest is reduced during REM sleep, or if the diaphragmatic contraction with significant airway restriction or obstruction exceeds the intercostal activity supporting the chest wall.[120] In Figure 5.7 Honma and associates illustrate that infants in non-rapid eye movement (NREM), or quiet sleep, have steady muscle tone in the intercostals, and there is coordinated breathing of chest and abdomen.[93] In rapid eye movement (REM) sleep, the breathing effort of the diaphragm pushes out the abdomen; but since there is a decrease in intercostal tone, the chest collapses inward reducing the size of the actual tidal volume by 20% to 50% or more. This is even more marked with complete airway obstruction.

5.3 *Definitions of Disturbed Ventilation*

Minute ventilation and the functional residual capacity will be reduced below the level that sustains arterial O_2 saturation, or clears carbon dioxide, with major decreases in ventilation frequency, regularity, or volume. A standard set of definitions for effective and ineffective breathing effort, hypopnea, reflex bradycardia, arterial hypoxia, hypercarbia, and the measurement of all three forms of apnea has been proposed.[121]

5.3.1　Apnea

Apnea is the absence of ventilation and is abnormally long if it exceeds 15 seconds. Shorter events, especially 10-12 seconds and less in duration, are commonly seen in most infants studied in sleep.[122]

Airflow may cease with:

Central apnea - absence or suppression of the signal stimulating the inspiratory muscles of respiration (Figure 5.8).

Obstructive apnea - respiratory effort without maintaining an open airway (Figure 5.9).

Mixed apnea - a single event composed of contiguous central apnea and intervals of obstruction or ineffective breaths (Figure 5.10).

Apnea is a common symptom seen with a number of primary conditions affecting infants, especially severe infections and following anesthesia in preterm infants who have reached 37 to 44 weeks post-conception.[122] It is also found as independent condition that frequently occurs with prematurity and a very small fraction of term infants experiencing an apparent life threatening event (ALTE) in the first months of life.[123] Treatment with

---

Figure 5.8— Central apnea during quiet sleep.

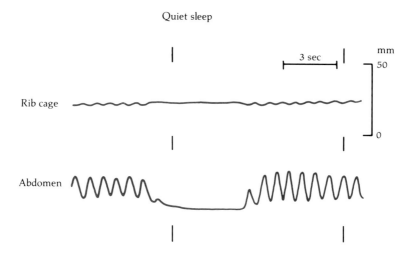

Figure 5.9— Obstructive apnea, 24 seconds long with all effort sensors failing to detect the change in airflow.

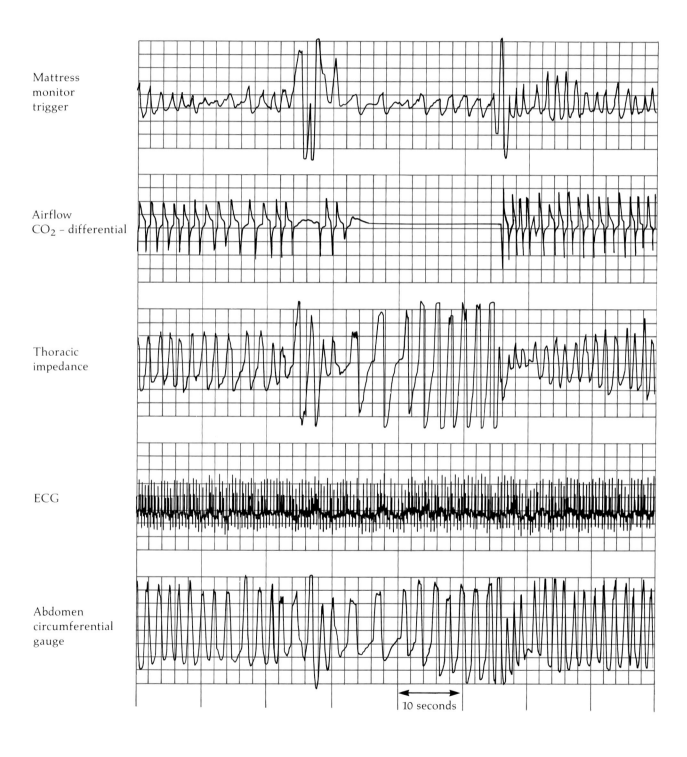

Figure 5.10— Mixed apnea: 18-second central apnea followed by 30 seconds of ineffectual and destructed effort.

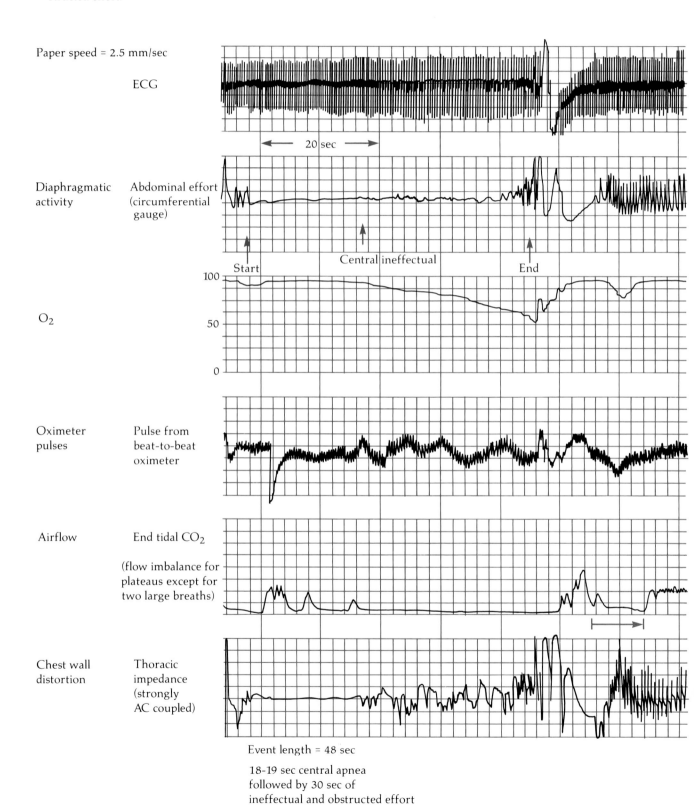

Paper speed = 2.5 mm/sec

ECG

← 20 sec →

Diaphragmatic activity — Abdominal effort (circumferential gauge)

Start   Central ineffectual   End

O₂   100   50   0

Oximeter pulses — Pulse from beat-to-beat oximeter

Airflow — End tidal CO₂

(flow imbalance for plateaus except for two large breaths)

Chest wall distortion — Thoracic impedance (strongly AC coupled)

Event length = 48 sec

18-19 sec central apnea followed by 30 sec of ineffectual and obstructed effort

medication and/or observation with monitors designed for home use are most commonly required for a few weeks after the presentation.[124] The goal is to confirm the gradual repair or maturation of breathing centers generating periods of defective breathing frequency under stress. This course is more severe and carries a greater risk of death if seizures or severe airway obstruction are part of the infant's pathophysiologic behavior.[125]

5.3.2 Periodic Breathing

Periodic breathing is composed of three or more central or mixed apneas 4 to 15 seconds long with each separated by no more than 20 seconds of stable regular breathing.[126] It is a frequent pattern in preterm infants and a third of normal term infants manifest short runs of periodic breathing in the first weeks after birth.[127] Periodic breathing is not seen in normal adults at sea level, but may occur with disturbed metabolic states such as ketoacidosis, anemia, or hypoxia.[128] It becomes increasingly common for mountain climbers sleeping at higher altitudes and while they are awake, at extreme altitude.[129] The pattern appears as a pathophysiologic change with progressive hypoxia and hypercarbia for a very small number of term infants (Figure 5.11), and a larger proportion of developing preterm infants approaching term post-conceptional ages.[130]

Periodic breathing is observed with residual lung disease after an acute pulmonary illness producing lung damage and is associated with very large fluctuations (30 to 40%) in breath-to-breath pulse O_2 level. There is also an elevated $ETCO_2$ plateau above 50 torr or mm Hg. The hypoxic drop in saturation is rapidly raised when the lung expands in the next cycle of breathing. This infant's periodic breathing disappeared with a low level of O_2 therapy. After an additional month of healing the same periodic breathing pattern produced no more than a 6% to 8% drop in breath-to-breath O_2 saturation. Use of a standard 5 to 6 second averaging interval would cause dampening of this oscillation and the oximeter would miss this pattern. Impedance monitors designed to detect prolonged runs of periodic breathing must accurately detect each short (4 to 15 second) breathing pause, and document breathing for the less than 20-second interval between pauses.

5.3.3 Hypopnea

The other important pattern of inadequate ventilation is hypopnea, or the inadequacy of ventilatory volumes with normal or near normal breathing frequency. Hypopnea (Figure 5.12) is the presence of breathing effort that is inadequate to clear arterial CO_2 at the rate produced, so that P_aCO_2 rises and arterial O_2 saturation usually falls. Primary hypopnea (Central Hypoventilation Syndrome) is detected at an early age in a very few individuals as a developmental defect or delay. There is a reduced breathing response to increased levels of CO_2 both when awake and, most markedly, in sleep.[131]

Hypopnea can also occur at a later age with any level of consciousness as the result of lung damage or muscle disease, and it again is most often worse in sleep.[132] This name implies deficiency in ventilation without total absence of ventilation for any sustained interval, and little or no evidence of obstruction. Often the respiratory rate is normal and the tidal volume is simply inadequate. Both the tidal volume and rate response to added inspired CO_2 during each level of sleep are usually present but inadequate.[133]

Hypopnea can only be detected by measuring minute ventilation, coupled with changes in CO_2 or O_2 that are sustained or progressively abnormal over minutes. Treatment usually requires a tracheostomy and artificial ventilation, or diaphragmatic pacing

Figure 5.11— Periodic breathing.

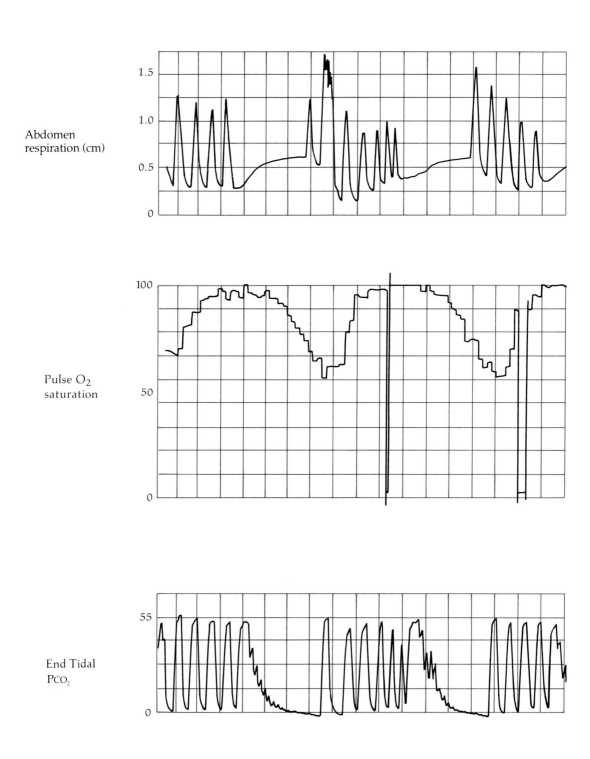

Abdomen respiration (cm)

Pulse O_2 saturation

End Tidal Pco_2

with sleep. Medical therapy is occasionally successful as well.[134] These invasive therapies are often needed to avoid life-threatening cardiopulmonary complications and possible sudden death in sleep.[135]

The transient shifts in CO_2 or O_2 following acute apneas are not usually long enough to be regarded as hypopnea. After many apneic events, the onset of breathing will be associated with elevated breathing rate and tidal volume suggesting an appropriate response to the CO_2 accumulation during the acute cessation of ventilation (Figure 5.10). By implication, the apnea for these patients may be caused by an overiding inhibitory signal that transiently suppresses normal breathing. Other patients appear to have more complex combined defects in both CO_2 response and pattern of breathing.[136]

5.4 *Limitations in Impedance Monitoring*

While thoracic impedance is widely used clinically there are a number of limitations in the signal that restrict its usefulness and precision.

5.4.1 **Physiologic Constraints**

As seen in Figure 5.4 and Table 5.2 the current between the two electrodes on the chest will follow a number of parallel paths with the greatest flow going through the tissues of lowest resistance. The blood and muscle layers of the chest wall, especially the large muscle groups over the back, represent the path of a large portion of the transmitted signal. Because of the extreme resistance of air, less than 1% of the base signal is estimated to traverse the lung to be influenced by the spacing and distortion of tissue fluid and blood volume reoriented by the entering air. Because air is extremely non-conductive there is no direct relationship to the air volume even in that small signal fraction.

Table 5.2—Tissues in the Chest Region Listed in Ascending Order According to Electrical Resistivity

Estimated Percent of Transmitted Signal	
Blood	45%
Muscle	35%
Bone	15%
Fat	5%
Air	1%

As described by the sequence seen during the animal experiment described in Section 5.1.3, the base signal and much of the variation in the respiration signal is virtually all due to changes in the volume and thickness of the pathways in blood, muscle and bone in the posterior chest wall, followed in significance by the anterior chest wall, the intrathoracic vessels, heart and blood forming a bridge through the lung, and lung tissue and air.[137]

Figure 5.12— Hyponea, the three segments reflect the breathing effort changes.

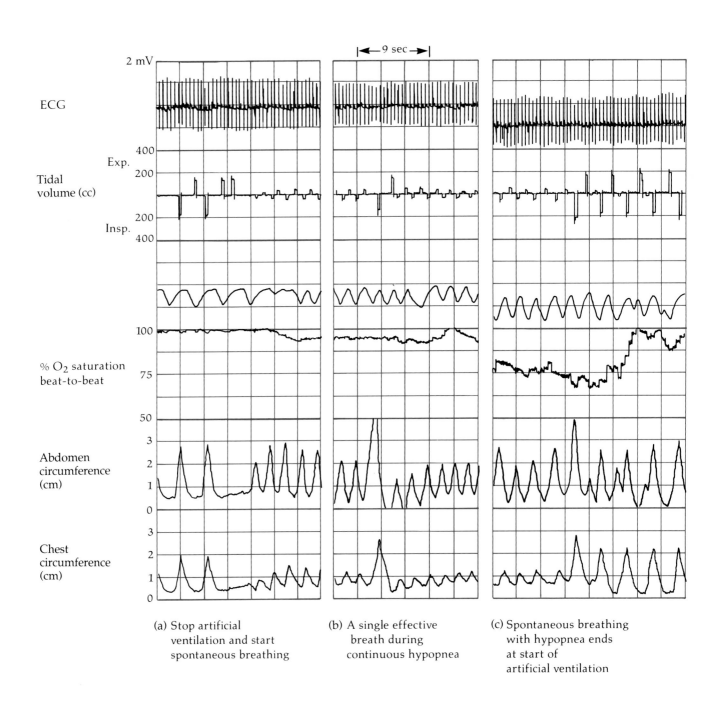

2 mV

|← 9 sec →|

ECG

Tidal volume (cc)

Exp.
400
200

Insp.
200
400

% O₂ saturation beat-to-beat
100
75
50

Abdomen circumference (cm)
3
2
1
0

Chest circumference (cm)
3
2
1
0

(a) Stop artificial ventilation and start spontaneous breathing

(b) A single effective breath during continuous hypopnea

(c) Spontaneous breathing with hypopnea ends at start of artificial ventilation

Figure 5.13— Two components of an infant cardiovascular artifact on impedance during quiet sleep.

ECG

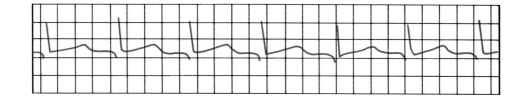

CVA
wave 1 = •
wave 2 = •

Thoracic
impedance

Ohms

1.5

1.0

0.5

0.0

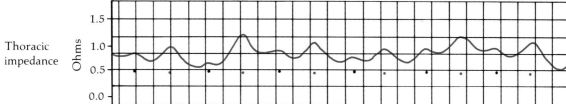

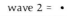

├────── 1 sec ──────┤

Abdomen
respiration
(Hg in silastic)

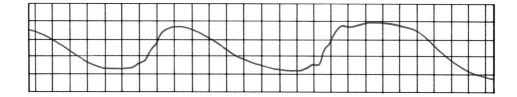

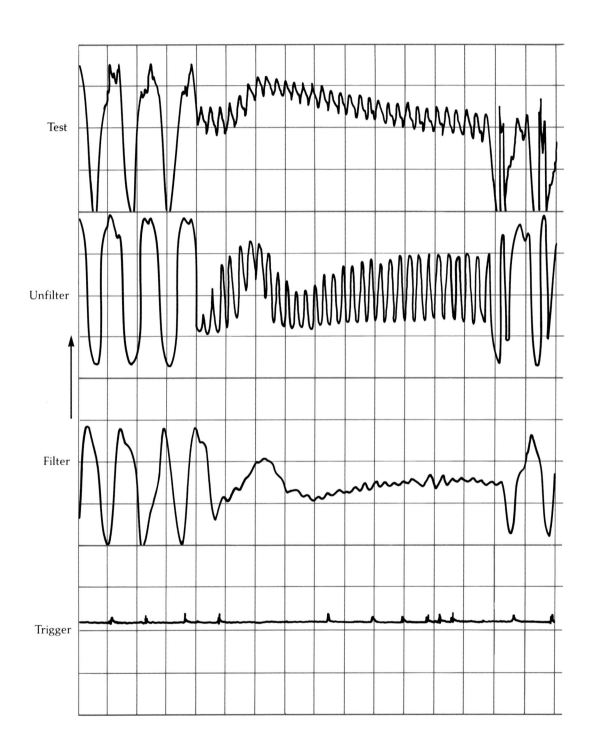

Figure 5.14— Central apnea lasting 20 seconds.

5.4.2   Cardiovascular Artifacts

Not only does the expansion and contraction of the chest cavity create impedance change, but so does the physical pumping of the heart and possibly the flow of blood through the vasculature of the chest, otherwise known as cardiovascular artifact. Clinically, a patient could be apneic, but a waveform representing impedance changes may still be present.

With the usual chest placement for electrodes, the depiction of the cardiovascular artifact is complicated by the fact that there are two components associated with each QRS complex (Figure 5.13). The illustration shows a segment of breathing in quiet sleep with minimal chest excursions and ample abdominal breathing. The cardiovascular artifact associated with each QRS interval is as large as the small thoracic signal showing breathing effort. Notice the two distinct components to each cardiovascular artifact. Wave 1 and wave 2 may change in relative dimension in our experience as a patient is moved from prone to supine position.[138] This implies that cardiac blood may not be a major source of the cardiovascular artifact.

It is possible that the two components of the cardiovascular signal superimposed on thoracic impedance may be due in large part to the dual peripheral arterial sources for blood flow to the chest wall, the mammary artery anteriorly and the vertebral arteries posteriorly. These two sources of flow may arrive out of phase and in different relative volumes at a chest skin site depending on supine or prone position of the patient. At the current time this is simply a speculation that explains the appearance of our data and the changes in signals associated with changing body position.

The acquisition device used to record the test signals shown in this section was linear from 0.01 Hz to 7.0 Hz, and as a result, accurately reproduced behavior not seen with most commercial equipment. A signal source similar to this would be needed in order to design and test monitors to be used for clinical purposes; however this type of unit has not always been available as a source of the test signals used by many manufacturers.

5.4.3   Signal Management

The ability to provide a useful estimate of breathing frequency is complicated by the multiple sources for signal variation with non-ventilating movements and cardiovascular activity. Figure 5.14 shows the failure of a respiration monitor to alarm for a prolonged apnea because of the false triggering of the respiration circuit on cardiac waves during central apnea.

Some monitors employ a filter to enhance detection of true apnea. Such filters watch for a coincidence of impedance waveforms and electrocardiographic activity. If the waveforms coincide for a specified number of heart beats, the monitor assumes the impedance waveform is actually due to cardiovascular artifact and the apnea alarm is activated. In cases where the patient's heart rate and respiratory rate are actually identical, the filter can be disabled.

There are no standards for the frequency response, precision, and reliability of signal reproduction, or even the polarity of voltages produced to represent changes in thoracic impedance. Because of apparent signal distortion, interference and suboptimal algorithms for detecting breathing and apnea, some currently distributed monitors detect 50% or less of carefully reproduced real central apnea events while producing false alarms at a high rate (>30/hour) during standardized testing procedures. Apnea alarm reliability among the 15 models tested and reported most recently was <10% apneas recognized for the worst to over 98%.[139]

5.4.4   Equipment Limitations

Independent of the physiologic limitations placed on the existing monitors, some equipment is not well suited to the task of detecting and displaying breathing activity because of compromises in design. There are no current standards for the electronics depicting thoracic impedance. This means that the signals created by each manufacturers circuit have unique limitations in displaying the occurence of breathing effort and in detecting breathing or apnea.

5.5   *Summary*

There are apparent differences in the degree of success that individual manufacturers have achieved in designing apnea alarms in current monitors. Some of the circuitry of early respiratory effort detecting devices has been shown to miss much or even most of the abnormal activity it was designed to detect.

Fortunately these commercial systems are continually being modified and improved, but at the this time the most recent effort to grade equipment response would suggest that the buyer of equipment for either the hospital or out-of-hospital market should understand its limitations. While thoracic impedance has been far from a perfect means of translating respiratory activity, much has been learned even with the limited methods at hand.

6.0   CAPNOGRAPHY AND GAS MONITORING

The lungs serve as the primary site for the elimination of carbon dioxide (CO_2) from the body. The CO_2 produced from metabolism is transported to the lungs and released during normal breathing. The lungs also offer an efficient route for drug administration, particularly in the operating room. Volatile anesthetic (inhalational) agents such as halothane, enflurane, and isoflurane can be administered by a vaporizer connected to the anesthesia circuit. The anesthetic agent is inhaled into the lungs and transferred to the blood stream as a result of the pressure gradient between the airways (alveoli) and the blood.

Because of the efficiency of the lungs in eliminating CO_2 and taking up anesthetic agents, monitoring the concentration of CO_2 capnography and anesthetic agents in the respiratory gases can provide the clinician with a reliable, noninvasive assessment of ventilation and anesthesia administered during surgery. These physiologic relationships provide the basis for respiratory gas monitoring. This section presents the principles of capnography and anesthetic gas monitoring and a description of the various technologies available to noninvasively monitor ventilation and anesthetic delivery.

6.1   *Capnography*

Capnography, which is the measurement of CO_2 tension in gas in the airways, was first introduced in 1975 by Smalhout and Kalenda. Since then it has become a routine method for evaluating the adequacy of ventilation in patients undergoing surgery. The technique can also be used to monitor ventilation of patients in the recovery room after surgery and in the intensive care unit. Capnography provides a direct measure of the CO_2 concentration in the gases going into and out of the lungs. The CO_2 level can be assessed during the entire respiratory cycle and then displayed digitally or as a waveform on an oscilloscope as CO_2 concentration versus time.

Capnography has several advantages over other ventilation monitoring techniques. It does not require a blood sample and therefore eliminates the risk of needle sticks and exposure of the health care worker to potentially contaminated blood. Capnography can be performed continuously, providing information about inspired and expired CO_2 concentration. The data can be displayed on an oscilloscope to provide the clinician with a graphic display (a capnograph) of CO_2 concentration or tension (partial pressure) over time. The information displayed can be used to evaluate the effectiveness of lung function. The instrument also provides a measure of the end-tidal partial pressure of CO_2 ($P_{ET}CO_2$), which is often a reliable estimate of the arterial CO_2 (P_aCO_2). Changes in CO_2 production ($\dot{V}CO_2$) can also be assessed by evaluating changes in $P_{ET}CO_2$ when the minute ventilation is constant.

A capnometer is an instrument that measures CO_2 levels in the lung during the respiratory cycle. The instrument can graphically display a waveform for the CO_2 concentration or tension (PCO_2) of gas in the airways during each breath. This graphic waveform display is known as a capnogram (Figure 6.1).

6.1.1   Gas Analysis

The carbon dioxide concentration in the airways of the lung can be measured using a number of technologies. The techniques currently available for clinical use include mass spectrometry, Raman spectrometry, and infrared (IR) absorption spectrophotometry.

6.1.1.1 Mass Spectrometry

Mass spectroscopy utilizes the relationship between the molecular charge and the mass of substances to determine their concentration. The mass spectrometer is a magnetic sector analyzer (Figure 6.2). It employs a sampling system to aspirate gas from the patient to the mass spectrometer. The gas sample diffuses into a high vacuum chamber in which an electrical field ionizes the sample into unique ion fragments. The ion fragments are then propelled through a magnetic field into a dispersion chamber where they separate according to mass and charge. The charged particles impact detector plates placed at specific locations that correspond to molecules of specific mass. The detector plates generate electric current. The total number of all plates impacted is proportional to the gas concentration.

For operating room use and other selected applications, mass spectroscopy is preferred because the technique allows monitoring of multiple respiratory gases in addition to CO_2. The mass spectrometer can monitor concentrations of O_2, CO_2, nitrogen, and volatile anesthetic agents (Section 6.2.1). The mass spectrometer is usually shared by multiple intrahospital sites, for example, operating rooms. It samples gas from each location sequentially, reporting the measured concentrations of the various gases and agents for each patient monitored.

The major advantages of mass spectrometry are its accuracy, response time, and ability to differentiate among multiple gases. The primary disadvantage of the mass spectrometer as a CO_2 monitor is that the instrument is generally shared among multiple hospital locations, samples gases intermittently, and does not provide a continuous record of

Figure 6.1— The normal capnogram.

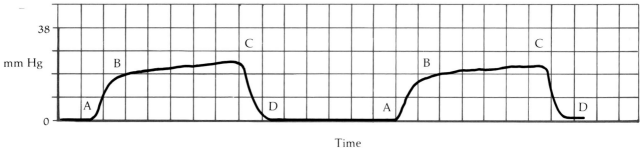

Figure 6.2— The mass spectrometer.

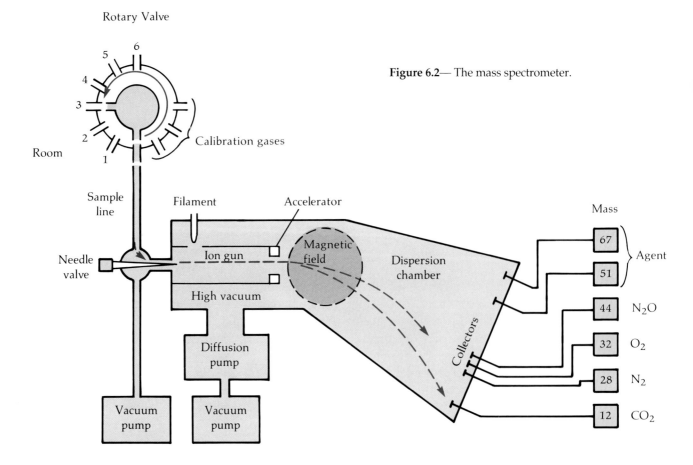

CO_2 concentration over time. These limitations undermine its value as a monitor of rapidly changing conditions, such as inappropriate endotracheal tube placement or a potential catastrophic cardiopulmonary event such as a pulmonary embolism which might occur in the operating room or intensive care unit. Mass spectrometers are also expensive to purchase and maintain and are not transportable. Another problem with this instrument is that nitrous oxide and CO_2 have nearly identical gram molecular weights, which could prevent specific identification of each compound. This difficulty is overcome by ionizing N_2O to N_2O^+ and ionizing CO_2 to CO_2^+.

6.1.1.2 Raman Spectrometry

Raman spectrometry uses the Raman effect to analyze the concentration of respiratory gases. Raman scattering occurs when photons from a laser beam collide with gas molecules. The collision between the light (photons) and the gas molecules slows down the photons, resulting in a change in color caused by an increase in wavelength. The change in frequency is specific to each molecule present in the sample. The wavelength shift and amount of scattering can be used to determine the constituents of a gas mixture.

A sample cell in commercially available systems based on Raman scattering contains 6 milliliters of gas. The instrument samples gas from the breathing circuit at 200 milliliters/minute. The sample cell is placed between the plasma tube and the output mirror of an air-cooled 40 mW argon laser. Lenses collect the scattered light while interference filters select Raman lines corresponding to the gases present in the cell. Raman scattering is not limited to polar gas species. Carbon dioxide, O_2, nitrogen, H_2O vapor, nitrous oxide, and volatile anesthetic agents all exhibit Raman activity. Photomultiplier tubes and a microcomputer produce simultaneous readings of the gas concentrations. A variety of types of laser have been used for Raman spectrometry, with argon lasers currently used in the commercially available Raman spectrometers.

Raman frequency shift peaks in wave numbers for the respiratory gases are as follows: CO_2 at 1285 and 1388 cm^{-1}, O_2 at 1555 cm^{-1}, nitrogen at 2331 cm^{-1}, and H_2O vapor at 3650 cm^{-1}. The size of the peaks at each of these frequencies gives an absolute measure of the concentration of the gas present in the sample cell.

Raman spectrometry is very efficient, although somewhat more expensive than other currently available technologies for measuring concentrations of CO_2 and anesthetic agents. The Raman scattering analyzer has some disadvantages when used in the clinical setting. The argon laser has a high power requirement and the laser source is expensive and has a limited life span. In an attempt to reduce the power needs and the cost associated with Raman spectrometers as well as to simplify the use of the instrument, lasers other than argon have been evaluated.

The Raman sample cell operates at approximately atmospheric pressure. It uses a sidestream sampling system which is affected by changes in the size and length of the sampling catheter and cuvette pressure. The method therefore does not work well if long sample tubing is required because of the pressure drop that occurs in long lines. The Raman analyzer is also sensitive to H_2O vapor in the sample cell because it measures cell partial pressure variation. The accuracy of the instrument is reduced as H_2O accumulates in the cell.

Figure 6.3—Infrared absorption spectra for carbon dioxide, water, and nitrous oxide.

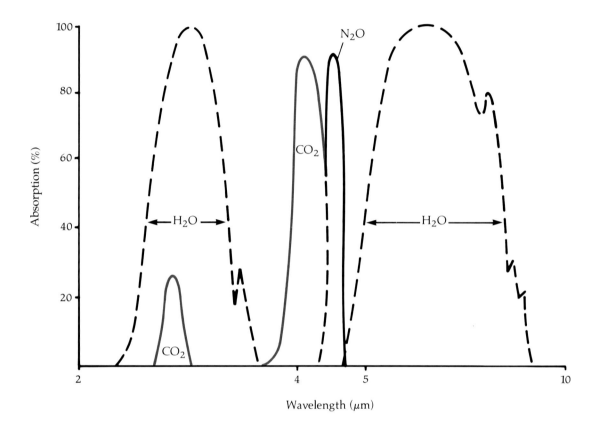

Figure 6.4— Nondispersive double-beam positive infrared capnometer.

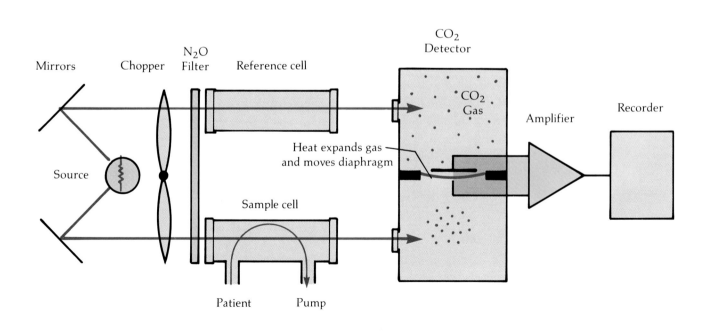

6.1.1.3   Infrared Spectrophotometry

Nondispersive infrared (IR) absorption spectrophotometry is the most frequently used method for monitoring CO_2 concentrations in the operating room, recovery room, and intensive care units. Infrared spectrophotometry employs the principle that different gases absorb infrared light at different wavelengths. Since CO_2 absorbs IR light at a known wavelength, the concentration of CO_2 can be determined using IR spectrophotometry. As a known spectrum of IR light passes through a gas sample, the amount of IR light absorbed is proportional to the concentration of CO_2 present in the sample. The amount of IR light absorbed by the CO_2 is compared to a known CO_2-free sample to calculate the amount of CO_2 present in the sample. The absorption peak for CO_2 is 4.26 micrometers. This absorption peak lies between the two IR absorption peaks for H_2O (Figure 6.3). The peaks for N_2O and carbon monoxide (CO) are so close to the peak for CO_2 that interference can occur. Another problem with the infrared capnometer is called pressure (or collision) broadening in which collisions between CO_2 and other gases affect the infrared energy absorption of CO_2. This problem can be overcome by applying known correction factors that adjust for the presence of gases other than CO_2.

Infrared capnometers use one of two techniques for analysis of gas contents. The nondispersive double-beam positive-filter capnometer has a reference cell, a sample cell, and a detector filled with CO_2 (Figure 6.4). Radiation that comes through the reference and sample cells affects the absorption of CO_2 in the detection chamber. The CO_2 in the sample cell decreases the radiation transmitted to the detector. The increased radiation transmitted from the reference cell compared to that transmitted from the sample cell produces movement of a diaphragm. The amount of movement of the diaphragm correlates with the amount of CO_2 present in the sample cell. Interference from N_2O is removed by a filter that absorbs radiation from the N_2O absorption band. A chopper periodically permits measurement of the reference signal, the sample signal and a dark signal, that is neither the reference nor sample signal.

A single-beam negative-filter capnometer directs an infrared signal through a sample cell to a detector, passing through a chopper wheel (Figure 6.5). The chopper wheel has two cells, one containing CO_2 and a second containing N_2. The ratio of the two detected signals is used to calculate the CO_2 concentration, a technique operating in mainstream capnometers (Section 6.1.2.1). With this technique, a sample chamber on the airway serves as a reference cell. During inspiration, the instrument assumes that CO_2-free gas is being inspired. In the presence of CO_2 rebreathing, this type of device does not provide an accurate measurement of CO_2.

A chopper is part of most infrared capnometers. For the double-beam capnometer, the chopper allows a common source and detector to be used. It also provides an alternating signal from the reference and sample cells. Finally, it produces a null signal from either the sample or reference cell to help eliminate drift and interference.

Many infrared capnometers require calibration at regular intervals. To calibrate the instruments, a gas mixture containing a known CO_2 concentration (usually 5% CO_2) is used. Most instruments must also undergo zero calibration with CO_2-free room air. The infrared capnometers should have an accuracy of ± 12% or ± 4 mm Hg (0.5 kPa). Some of the newer infrared capnometers do not require user calibration.

Figure 6.5— Single-beam negative-filter infrared capnometer.

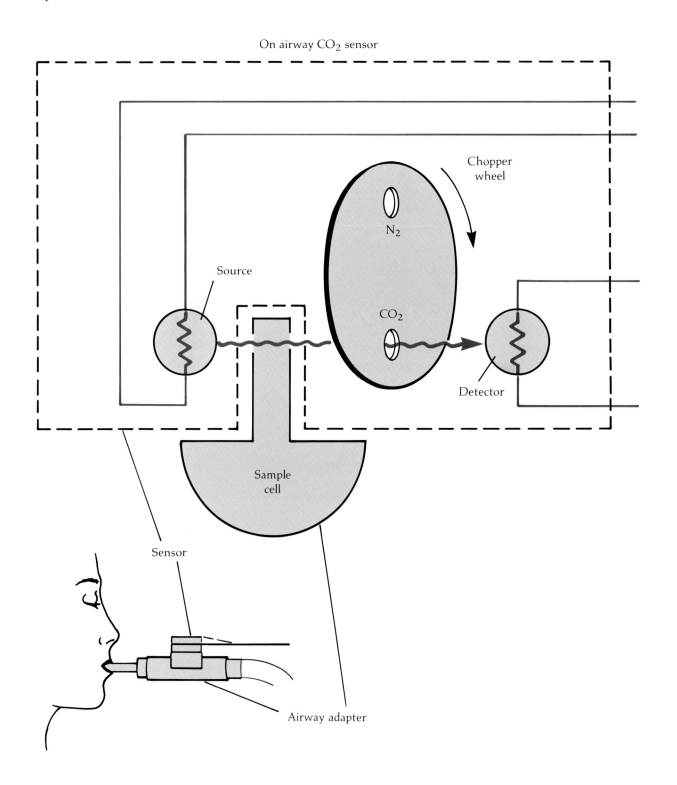

On airway CO$_2$ sensor

Chopper wheel

N$_2$

CO$_2$

Source

Detector

Sample cell

Sensor

Airway adapter

Figure 6.6— Mainstream capnometer. (a) diagrammatic relationship of the components of a mainstream capnometer; (b) schematic representation of airway adaptor and CO_2 transducer.

(a) Components of a mainstream caprometer

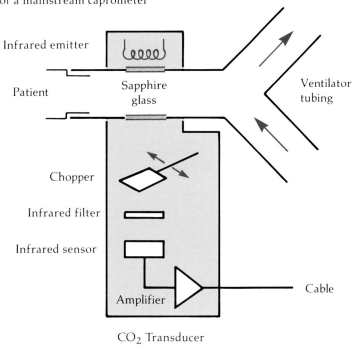

CO$_2$ Transducer

(b) Airway adaptor and CO_2 transducer

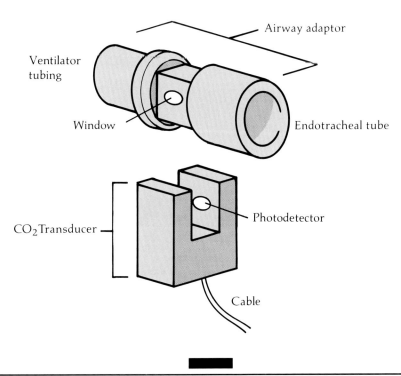

Figure 6.7— Sidestream capnometer.

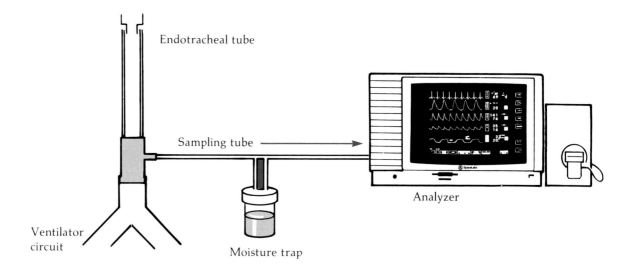

Endotracheal tube

Sampling tube

Analyzer

Ventilator
circuit

Moisture trap

6.1.2   Gas Sampling Techniques

Capnometers analyze the concentration of CO_2 in the gas sample using one of two sampling techniques: either the mainstream (in-line) within an airway adaptor in the breathing circuit, or the sidestream (diverting) technique in which a sample of gas is aspirated into the capnometer where the gas concentrations are measured.

6.1.2.1   Mainstream Capnometers

Mainstream analyzers use a transducer located on an airway connector placed in the patient breathing circuit (Figure 6.6). The mainstream instruments generate a capnogram almost immediately. The transducer contains both the IR light source and a photodetector, which must be heated to approximately 40 degrees centigrade to prevent condensation from accumulating on its window. Since the analysis of the gas concentration occurs in the airway adaptor, mainstream capnographs have a rapid response time, often under one-half second.

　　The airway connectors for mainstream capnometers are relatively large and heavy, adding as much as 15 milliliters of dead space and 2 to 3 ounces of weight to the patient's airway with the transducer in place. Transducers have to be carefully supported to prevent the endotracheal tube from kinking or becoming dislodged. They also must be handled with care to prevent damage to the light source or photodetector. The mainstream sampling technique cannot be used in nonintubated patients.

6.1.2.2   Sidestream Capnometers

The sidestream capnometer, also called an aspirating or diverting capnometer, withdraws gas from the patient's airway through narrow bore tubing to a sample-measuring chamber inside the capnometer. A sampling tube, free of leaks and impermeable to CO_2, and an aspirating system are required to actively aspirate gas to the capnometer (Figure 6.7). The sampling tube must have a small internal diameter, usually no greater than 2 millimeters to allow for rapid, linear withdrawal of gas without creating turbulence. Gas analysis occurs in the capnometer, which contains the light source and a photodetector. The sampling for a mass spectrometer employs a sidestream sampling technique.

　　Because the gas samples must be aspirated to the instrument, the transit time between the initiation of gas sampling in the airway and the detection of the gas by the analyzer can take as long as 2 to 3 seconds. The major determinant of the response time in sidestream analyzers is the sampling flow rate (SFR), the rate at which gas is aspirated from the airway to the instrument. Most sidestream capnographs have SFRs of 50 to 150 milliliters/minute. The use of a flow that is too low results in artifact in the capnographic waveform. When using a sidestream capnometer, the aspirating tubing must be positioned carefully to prevent air entrapment, which would contaminate the sample. When a sidestream device is used in the operating room, the capnometer must be equipped with a scavenging system to prevent contamination of the operating room environment with aspirated anesthetic gases.

　　The gas sampling from a sidestream analyzer can be affected by H_2O condensation or airway secretions that accumulate in the sampling tube. These liquids can interrupt the flow of gas to the capnograph, producing an inaccurate measurement of CO_2 concentration. To prevent excess contamination from H_2O and secretions, sidestream

Figure 6.8— Capnogram with alveolar (curare) cleft. The cleft in the alveolar plateau represents inspiratory effort by the patient due to ineffective diaphragmatic activity.

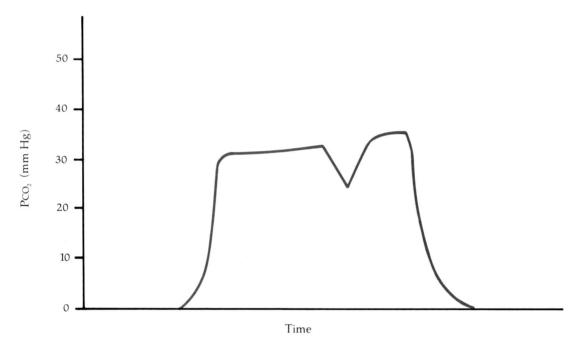

Figure 6.9— Capnogram of a patient with severe airflow obstruction due to bronchospasm. The expiratory phases is prolonged and the capnogram lacks an alveolar plateau, indicating that alveolar emptying is inadequate.

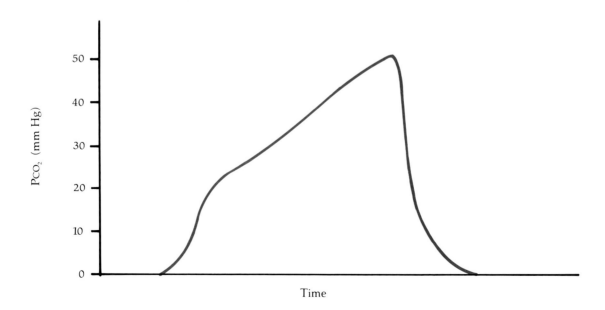

capnometers utilize H_2O traps and a filter. Water-permeable Nalfion® tubing is also used by some manufacturers. Some instruments employ reverse flow or purge systems to remove excess H_2O or mucus from the sampling line.

Infrared spectrophotometry is relatively inexpensive and simple to use, particularly for measurement of CO_2. The technique has been well-tested in the clinical environment and has been readily accepted by clinicians. The instruments are easily transportable and easily calibrated.

6.1.3 The Normal Capnogram

The normal capnogram is illustrated in Figure 6.1. It has four components: the baseline, ascending limb, alveolar plateau, and descending limb. As exhalation begins (Figure 6.1, point A), the gas in the initial sample contains no CO_2 since it is the gas coming from airways which are not involved in gas exchange. The steep ascending limb (Figure 6.1, segment A-B) represents the CO_2 concentration that is in the gas emptying the alveoli, the lung units in which gas exchange occurs. The CO_2 concentration remains relatively stable during this phase of exhalation (the alveolar plateau phase) (Figure 6.1, segment B-C) while gases from uniformly ventilated areas of the lung are exhaled. The end tidal CO_2 concentration ($P_{ET}CO_2$) is the point where the CO_2 concentration is usually the highest (Figure 6.1, point C), representing the gas in the alveoli (P_aCO_2) which most closely approximates the arterial CO_2 tension (P_aCO_2). The beginning of inspiration is signaled by the rapid descent on the waveform (Figure 6.1, segment C-D). Since inspired gas should contain no CO_2, a baseline PCO_2 of 0 mm Hg will be measured, unless CO_2 rebreathing is occurring.

The normal capnogram demonstrates a nearly constant PCO_2 during the plateau phase (Figure 6.1, segment B-C). The alveolar plateau is flat because the expired gas from all lung units have similar relationships between ventilation and perfusion of the lung. If the patient has significant maldistribution of ventilation, exhaled gas from various parts of the lung will have differing concentrations of CO_2, since the CO_2 concentration from some airways will be low (representing dead space ventilation), while the CO_2 concentration from others will be high. In this situation the CO_2 waveform will have a slow, rising expiratory upstroke and may have no alveolar plateau (Figure 6.9). For the $P_{ET}CO_2$ to represent the true alveolar CO_2 concentration, the capnogram must have a distinct alveolar plateau.

6.1.4 Clinical Applications of Capnography

6.1.4.1 Clinical Utility

The capnogram and $P_{ET}CO_2$ are useful monitors of the adequacy of ventilation and ventilation/perfusion relationships and provide an indication of the CO_2 production ($\dot{V}CO_2$). Capnography, therefore, aids in monitoring patients in the operating room, recovery room, and in the intensive care units—to monitor healthy patients undergoing elective surgical procedures as well as critically-ill patients with respiratory failure. Capnography provides valuable physiologic information and serves as an invaluable safety monitor of ventilation. This technique can confirm the correct placement of an endotracheal tube, assess the appropriateness of mechanical ventilatory support, and provide information about a patient's ability to tolerate weaning from mechanical ventilation and the presence of significant obstructive airways disease. Capnography can indicate when a patient is rebreathing expired CO_2 due to a faulty ventilator circuit or inadequate fresh gas flow. It has recently been used to monitor perfusion during cardiopulmonary resuscitation and may help determine the appropriate timing of hemodynamic pressure measurements.

6.1.4.2　Endotracheal Tube Positioning

The documentation of proper endotracheal tube placement can be confirmed by the presence of CO_2 in the expired gases. If the esophagus is intubated accidentally or the properly-placed endotracheal tube becomes dislodged, the $P_{ET}CO_2$ will suddenly drop to zero and the capnogram waveform disappear, since the CO_2 concentration in the stomach should approximate that in air. In cases of accidental placement of the endotracheal tube too far into the trachea, resulting in an endobronchial intubation, a capnogram will be noted, but the $P_{ET}CO_2$ will be lower than expected.

Capnography is also a useful monitor of endotracheal tube integrity and positioning after initial placement. An abnormal capnogram will result if the endotracheal tube becomes kinked or obstructed. If the endotracheal tube becomes partially obstructed, (for example with thick pulmonary secretions), the CO_2 waveform will develop a slow, expiratory upstroke. Endotracheal tube cuff leaks can also be detected. The $P_{ET}CO_2$ concentration will be low because some of the exhaled gas leaks around the endotracheal tube and the CO_2 in that gas is not detected by the capnograph. If the patient is accidentally extubated, either because of a vigorous cough or as a result of a position change, the $P_{ET}CO_2$ value will suddenly drop as happens when the endotracheal tube is accidentally inserted into the esophagus.

6.1.4.3　Mechanical Ventilation

The capnogram provides useful continuous, noninvasive data about adequacy of ventilation in patients who require mechanical ventilatory support during surgery or in the intensive care unit. The $P_{(a-ET)}CO_2$ gradient ($P_aCO_2 - P_{ET}CO_2$) can be used as a guide to titrate and determine the best level of positive end-expiratory pressure (PEEP) to use for those patients who have poor oxygenation. The capnograph can also provide useful information about the return of diaphragmatic function after the administration of neuromuscular blocking drugs to patients in the operating room or intensive care unit. The presence of a negative cleft in the alveolar plateau (curare cleft) indicates partial return of muscle function (Figure 6.8). The cleft reflects diaphragmatic contraction.

For a patient being mechanically ventilated using the assist control mode of ventilation, an inappropriate sensitivity setting can be diagnosed with the capnogram. If the sensitivity is set too high, spontaneous respiratory efforts generate a negative airway pressure that fails to result in a ventilator-assisted breath. The capnogram reveals a cleft during the alveolar plateau similar to that represented in Figure 6.8.

The capnogram can diagnose and monitor maldistribution of ventilation during mechanical ventilation. In patients who have lung units with abnormal ventilation/perfusion relationships, the capnogram can have a steeper slope throughout the expiratory phase and lose the normal alveolar plateau defined in Figure 6.1. The capnogram for patients with bronchospasm, for example, may not have a normal alveolar plateau because the alveoli are not emptying completely before the next breath is initiated. The capnogram will then have a steep slope, as illustrated in Figure 6.9. When this occurs, the measured $P_{ET}CO_2$ does not provide a good estimate of P_aCO_2. The slope of the expiratory phase on the capnogram can be monitored during treatment with bronchodilating drugs. As bronchospasm (wheezing) resolves, the slope of the expiratory phase becomes less steep and an alveolar plateau returns, suggesting improvement in the distribution of ventilation.

Changes in CO_2 production ($\dot{V}CO_2$) can be determined by monitoring the $P_{ET}CO_2$. Acute increases in $P_{ET}CO_2$ can occur in a variety of clinical situations, particularly when the patient is sedated or paralyzed and not able to increase minute ventilation. An increase in CO_2 production occurs after administration of sodium bicarbonate as during CPR, during rewarming after surgical procedures performed using cardiopulmonary bypass, malignant hyperthermia, and during removal of pneumatic antishock garments. When CO_2 production increases, the $P_{ET}CO_2$ provides immediate and direct data with which to adjust ventilatory parameters to optimize the P_aCO_2 and prevent complications.

6.1.4.4 Weaning from Mechanical Ventilation

Capnography provides useful information about the patient's ventilatory status during weaning from mechanical ventilatory support. A rising $P_{ET}CO_2$ and/or loss of a good alveolar plateau on the capnogram usually represents a failing weaning attempt. The capnographic waveform can also produce useful information about the development of significant bronchospasm or gas trapping that can occur during weaning trials. The increase in airway resistance in this situation is manifested by a slow expiratory upstroke on the capnogram.

The shape of sequential capnograms can indicate the status of the patient being weaned from ventilatory support by synchronized intermittent mandatory ventilation (SIMV). Patients with normal lungs have a similar capnogram from breath to breath despite varying tidal volumes that might be taken during SIMV. Patients with significant lung disease, however, often have marked variations in tidal volume and expiratory time, causing varying and inadequate alveolar plateaus from breaths taken spontaneously versus those provided by the ventilator (Figure 6.10).

6.1.4.5 Carbon Dioxide Rebreathing

For patients requiring ventilatory support, rebreathing of exhaled CO_2 can occur, particularly if the O_2 delivery system does not have an adequate fresh gas flow. The capnograph can provide a visual indication of CO_2 rebreathing. If a patient begins to rebreathe gas containing CO_2, the inspired CO_2 tension rises above zero and may continue to rise with each successive breath (Figure 6.11).

Figure 6.10— Capnogram from a patient ventilated with synchronized intermittent mandatory ventilation (SIMV), demonstrating the capnogram obtained during a ventilated breath (a) and from a spontaneous breath (b).

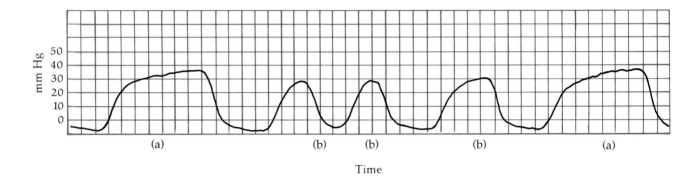

Figure 6.11— Capnogram from a patient who is rebreathing CO_2.

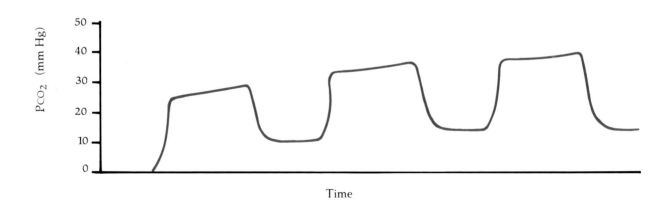

Rebreathing of CO_2 can occur in the critically-ill patient for a number of reasons. The patient rebreathes expired gas containing CO_2 if the expiratory valve is dislodged or missing from a self-inflating resuscitation bag. If the fresh gas flow provided to a t-piece ventilating system is less than about two times the minute ventilation, rebreathing of expired gas occurs. An incompetent expiratory valve in the ventilator circuit also causes rebreathing.

6.1.4.6 Cardiopulmonary Resuscitation

Capnography is useful during cardiopulmonary resuscitation (CPR). The $P_{ET}CO_2$ falls precipitously following cessation of perfusion after cardiac arrest. As the output from the heart ceases, pulmonary blood flow falls and CO_2 is no longer eliminated by the lung because the blood containing the high CO_2 does not reach the lungs for exhalation. As the patient is resuscitated, systemic and pulmonary blood flow return and CO_2 can be eliminated by the lung. The capnogram becomes a helpful noninvasive monitor of the adequacy of perfusion during CPR, particularly during closed chest cardiac compressions. It also provides a useful prognostic indicator of survival after CPR. Patients who can be successfully resuscitated have an increase in $P_{ET}CO_2$ during CPR, while those not resuscitated continue to have a low $P_{ET}CO_2$ despite closed chest resuscitation.

6.1.4.7 Hemodynamic Monitoring

The accurate determination of pulmonary artery (PA) pressures and the pulmonary capillary wedge pressure can be very difficult and can be inaccurate in some critically ill patients, particularly for those breathing rapidly with a great deal of respiratory variation in the PA pressures measured. The capnogram can aid in the timing of hemodynamic measurements to end-expiration. If the capnogram and PA pressure waveform are synchronized, the timing of end-expiration can be accurately determined and the pressure measurements reliably obtained (Figure 6.12). This technique may only be possible with mainstream capnographs, since an inherent time delay is associated with sidestream capnographs. Formal clinical studies are necessary to confirm this relationship and to document the value of mainstream capnography in facilitating the determination of end-expiration to guide the measurement of hemodynamic parameters.

6.1.4.8 Use for Monitoring Nonintubated Patients

Capnometers can monitor ventilation in spontaneously breathing, nonintubated patients. Sidestream analyzers equipped with specially-adapted nasal cannulae can sample expired gas and measure the CO_2 concentration. The cannulae are modified so that gas sampling occurs through one port and O_2 delivery through the other (Figure 6.13). The data obtained with these devices can be very useful, but must be interpreted with caution. The accuracy of $P_{ET}CO_2$ measurement in the spontaneously breathing patient depends on the proper placement of the sampling tube in the patient's nare, or nasopharyngeal airway. If the patient exhales through the mouth, the $P_{ET}CO_2$ measured will not reflect the true $P_{ET}CO_2$.

Figure 6.12— Synchronized recording of pulmonary artery (PA) pressure and pulmonary capillary wedge pressure measurements (upper waveform) and the capnogram from a mainstream capnometer (lower waveform). The arrow indicates the end-expiratory point on the capnogram to assist in the determination of the pulmonary capillary wedge pressure in a patient who has significant respiratory variation in the PA pressure waveform.

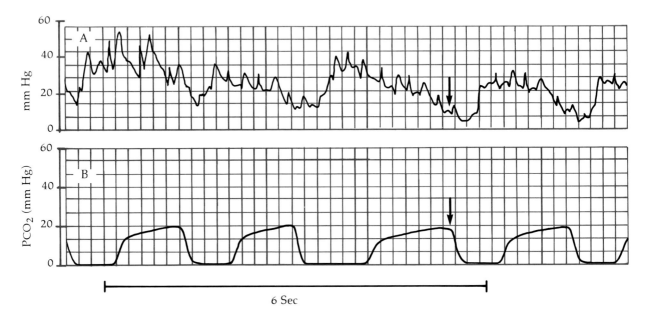

6 Sec

Figure 6.13— Modified nasal cannulae used in monitor CO_2 using a sidestream capnometer while simultaneously providing supplemental oxygen.

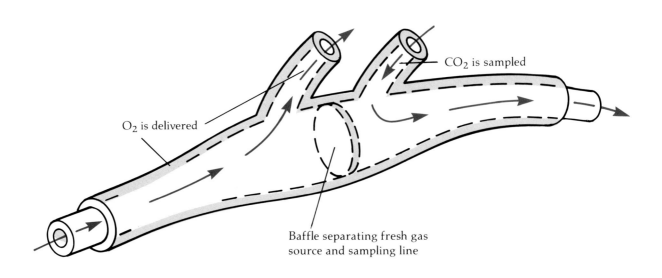

O_2 is delivered

CO_2 is sampled

Baffle separating fresh gas source and sampling line

6.1.5   Limitations of Capnography

Capnography has a number of limitations. When used to monitor ventilation in some patients with severe respiratory failure, the relationship between the $P_{ET}CO_2$ and P_aCO_2 can be poor. In addition, not only can the correlation between these values be low, but the $P_{(a-ET)}CO_2$ gradient can vary over time in an individual patient. Even in the normal person without significant lung disease, the relationship between P_aCO_2 and $P_{ET}CO_2$ can vary over time. Some studies evaluating the relationship between $P_{ET}CO_2$ and P_aCO_2 in patients being weaned from ventilatory support have shown a poor correlation between these parameters. The $P_{ET}CO_2$ measurements, therefore, must be correlated with P_aCO_2 measurements regularly. The $P_{ET}CO_2$ values and the capnographic waveform are supplements to, rather than replacements for, P_aCO_2 values.

6.1.6   Capnography Summary

Capnometers are commercially available as stand-alone units or as a modular component for a multiparameter bedside monitor. Modular instruments have the advantage of the respiratory data being integrated with hemodynamic and electrocardiographic data on a single display. Infrared instruments are often combined with pulse oximeters, noninvasive blood pressure monitors, or other monitoring devices into a freestanding and portable device.

When selecting an instrument, the sampling technique should be carefully considered. The choice of a mainstream or sidestream device depends on the importance of monitoring nonintubated patients and on concerns about the response time of the instruments. The sidestream device can be used to monitor nonintubated patients, while the mainstream device cannot. The response time for the sidestream instruments is slower than that for the mainstream capnographs. For the intubated patient, the weight and deadspace of the mainstream device is of concern, particularly in the intensive care unit when used to monitor patients who are alert and mobile. When selecting a sidestream analyzer, the adequacy of the moisture control system must be taken into account, including the mechanisms that control moisture and prevent secretions from occluding the sampling tube.

6.2   *Anesthetic Agent Monitoring*

In the operating room, the monitoring of concentrations of volatile, inhalational anesthetic agents has become routine. This monitoring technique assures that the correct agent is administered and that the concentration provided to the patient is appropriate. It also guarantees that the delivery system for the vaporizers used to vaporize the liquid anesthetic agent is working properly.

Ultraviolet spectrophotometry, silicone rubber elasticity, quartz crystal oscillation, mass spectroscopy, Raman scattering, and infrared spectrometry have all been used to assess the concentration of anesthetic agents. The most popular techniques currently in use include mass spectrometry, Raman spectrophotometry, and infrared spectrophotometry. Other techniques, such as an acoustic technology using lasers, have been used to monitor the concentration of anesthetic agents in respiratory gases.

6.2.1   Mass Spectrometry

Mass spectrometry can assess inspired and expired volatile anesthetic agent concentrations in the operating room using the same technique as is used to monitor CO_2 (Section 6.1.1.1). Gas is aspirated into an instrument located away from the operating room. The gas sample is analyzed with a magnetic sector analyzer, differentiating agents based on their mass-charge ratio. The instruments are shared among a number of operating rooms, typically up to ten rooms. The instrument can differentiate each anesthetic agent used, so that, if more than one agent were accidently administered, the clinician would observe specific concentrations of each agent.

The mass spectrometer has a number of advantages as an anesthetic agent monitor. The technique is very accurate, has a rapid response time so that changes in the inspired or expired anesthetic agent levels are immediately reflected in the measurement, and can distinguish among the many anesthetic agents. The mass spectrometer can also monitor nitrogen levels in respiratory gases, which is used to determine if air has been introduced into the breathing circuit, from a ventilator circuit disconnection or leak, or that the patient has an air embolus. This technique of checking for air emboli is the most sensitive and specific. By early detection, the patient can be rapidly treated and serious consequences of air emboli avoided.

The major disadvantages of mass spectrometers used to monitor anesthetic agents are the high cost, large maintenance requirements, and the need to share the instrumentation with other operating rooms. The shared technology prevents rapid reporting of changes in anesthetic concentration and does not provide continuous CO_2 monitoring or monitoring of nitrogen. Since most clinicians prefer continuous CO_2 monitoring, many operating rooms using mass spectrometers for anesthetic agent monitoring utilize other instrumentation, such as infrared spectrometers, to assess CO_2.

6.2.2   Raman Spectrometry

Raman spectrophotometry is currently available to monitor specific anesthetic agents in addition to CO_2 concentrations in respiratory gases. For CO_2 monitoring, an argon laser light source is used (Section 6.1.1.2). The anesthetic gas concentrations are proportional to the amount of light at the different wavelengths. Raman spectrometry provides a reliable measure of the specific anesthetic agent being administered. The advantages of this technology for many anesthesiologists include its relatively simple operation, lower cost compared to mass spectrometry, and lower maintenance. The argon laser, however, has a limited life span and the power requirements of the instrument are high. Other lasers have been evaluated to address these concerns, but none are ready for clinical use.

Raman optical signals provided by anesthetic agents administered at concentrations of about 1% as used clinically are rather weak and may overlap. The noise level for these instruments is therefore large: for example, noise levels of ±0.13% for halothane and ±0.05% for isoflurane are significantly greater than those for a mass spectrometer with a typical noise level as low as ±0.02%. The Raman scattering analyzer also calibrates only with an argon-free background and room air nitrogen and O_2 peaks. The instrument does not provide any calibration for CO_2 or anesthetic agents whose strength ratios relative to nitrogen and O_2 are assumed to remain constant.

6.2.3   Infrared Spectrophotometry

Infrared spectrophotometry is used to measure levels of anesthetic agents as well as CO_2 (Section 6.1.1.3). The principle in that technique is the different gases absorb infrared light at different wavelengths. Most clinical systems are optical, using a photodetector to determine amount of light transmitted after the light passes through the gas sample. The advantages of infrared spectrometry to other techniques are that it is inexpensive, simple to use, and reliable in the clinical environment.

Infrared spectrophotometry has a number of disadvantages for monitoring volatile anesthetic agents. First, nitrogen and O_2 have no infrared absorption spectrum. To measure these gases, an alternate method is required. Many of the commercially available infrared monitors cannot differentiate specific anesthetic agents. The monitor provides information about the concentration of the agent administered, but the user must identify which specific agent is being used. In addition, several chambers are required to assess all gases being monitored. This complicates the technique and makes it difficult to measure all gases simultaneously.

6.3   *Summary*

Monitoring the concentration of CO_2 and anesthetic agents from respiratory gases in the intensive care unit and operating room has become common place. The techniques today are reliable, cost-effective, and have significantly improved the safety of anesthesia in the operating room and of ventilation in the recovery room and intensive care units. The available techniques provide useful, noninvasive, and continuous monitors of ventilation with minimal risk. The American Society of Anesthesiologists, the Society of Critical Care Medicine, and many legislative bodies recognize the value of these monitoring methods and have either recommended or mandated their use. The clinical applications for capnography, particularly in the intensive care environment and in the nonintubated patient, are expected to increase as better monitors are designed and the understanding of the physiology of capnography increases. Additional studies, however, must confirm that capnography and agent-specific anesthesia monitoring actually improve patient outcome and reduce the costs of caring for patients in the operating room, recovery room, and intensive care units.

7.0   ABBREVIATIONS

Note: For oxygenation/ventilation measurements, the <u>capital</u> letters indicate the physical quantities and secondary symbol indicates the location of the measurement.

A slash (-) over a symbol denotes mixed or mean value

A dot (.) over a symbol indicates a unit of time

a	arterial
A	area or alveolar
a/A	arterial alveolar ratio
AC	alternating current
A/D	analog to digital
Ag	silver
A-P	anterior-posterior
Au	gold
C	compliance
C_aO_2	oxygen content of arterial blood
$C_{\bar{v}}O_2$	oxygen content of venous blood
$C_{(a-\bar{v})}O_2$	arterial-venous oxygen content difference
c' flow	end-pulmonary capillary blood flow
CI	cardiac index
Cl	chloride
cm	centimeter
CO	carbon monoxide or cardiac output
CO_2	carbon dioxide
COHb	carboxyhemoglobin
CO_2	oxygen content in blood
CPR	cardiopulmonary resuscitation
D	diffusion
DC	direct current
dl	deciliter
DO_2	oxygen delivery
e^-	electron
E	elasticity or energy or voltage
ERV	expiratory reserve volume
ET	end-tidal
$ETCO_2$	end-tidal carbon dioxide
ETO_2	end-tidal oxygen
f	breathing or respiratory frequency
F	fahrenheit
FEF	forced expiratory flow
F_EO_2	fractional concentration of expired oxygen

FEV	forced expiratory volume
FiO_2	fractional inspired oxygen concentration
F_IO_2	fractional concentration of inspired oxygen
FRC	functional residual capacity
ft	feet
gm	gram
H^+	hydrogen ion
H_2	hydrogen
Hb	hemoglobin
HCO_3^-	bicarbonate ion
H_2CO_3	carbonic acid
H_2O	water
He	helium
Hg	mercury
Hz	hertz
ICU	intensive care unit
in	inches
IPPB	intermittent positive pressure breathing
IR	infrared
IRV	inspiratory reserve volume
k	constant
kg	kilogram
kPa	kiloPascal
L	length
l	liters
lb	pound
LED	light-emitting diode
LPM(l/min)	liters per minute
M	mass
mM	millimoles
mm	millimeters
mW	milliwatt
MAP	mean arterial pressure
MetHb	methemoglobin
ml	milliliters
min	minute
MW	molecular weight
n	mass or number of gas molecules

NICU	neonatal intensive care unit
N_2	nitrogen
N_2O	nitrous oxide
nm	nanometer
OH^-	hydroxyl ions
O_2	oxygen
P	pressure
P_a	arterial pressure
P_v	venous pressure
P_A	alveolar pressure
P_B	barometric pressure
PH_2O	water vapor pressure
PN_2	nitrogen pressure
PO_2	oxygen partial pressure
P_aCO_2	arterial carbon dioxide partial pressure
P_aO_2	arterial oxygen partial pressure
P_ACO_2	alveolar carbon dioxide partial pressure
P_AO_2	alveolar oxygen partial pressure
P_cCO_2	capillary carbon dioxide partial pressure
P_cO_2	capillary oxygen partial pressure
$P_{ET}CO_2$	end-tidal partial pressure of CO_2
PIO_2	inspired oxygen partial pressure
PCO_2	mixed venous carbon dioxide partial pressure
PO_2	mixed venous oxygen partial pressure
$P_{(A-a)}O_2$	alveolar-arterial oxygen gradient
$P_{(a-ET)}CO_2$	arterial-end tidal carbon dioxide gradient
$P_{(I-E)}O_2$	oxygen partial pressure gradient between inspired and end-tidal gas
pH	a measure of acidity or alkalinity of a solution
ΔP	pressure change
PA	pulmonary artery
PAOP	pulmonary artery occlusion pressure
Pb	lead
PEEP	positive end-expiratory pressure
PSI	pounds per square inch (pressure)
Pt	platinum
PVC	premature ventricular contraction
r	radius
R	gas constant or resistance

ΔR	resistive change in impedance
RAM	random access memory
REM	rapid eye movement
RV	residual volume
$\dot{Q}$	blood flow
$\dot{Q}sp$	physiological shunt
$\dot{Q}sp/\dot{Q}t$	intrapulmonary shunt fraction
SaO_2	arterial oxygen saturation
SaO_2 frac	fractional arterial oxygen saturation
SaO_2 func	functional arterial oxygen saturation
$Sc'O_2$	oxygen saturation of the end-pulmonary capillary
sec	second
SFR	sampling flow rate
SIMV	synchronized intermittent mandatory ventilation
$S\bar{v}O_2$	mixed venous oxygen saturation
SpO_2	pulse oximetry arterial oxygen saturation
T	temperature
t	thickness
Te	expiratory cycle time
Ti	inspiratory cycle time
torr	1 mm Hg
υ	viscosity
$\dot{V}_E$	minute ventilation
$\dot{V}$	gas flow
V	volume
$\dot{V}_{gas}$	rate of transfer (diffusion) of a gas
ΔV	volume change
$\dot{V}_D$	minute deadspace ventilation
V_D	deadspace gas
$\bar{v}$	mixed venous blood
$\dot{V}_A$	minute alveolar ventilation
V/Q	ventilation/perfusion ratio
V_A	alveolar gas volume
V_D/V_T	dead space to tidal volume ratio
vol%	volumes percent
V_T	tidal volume
$\dot{V}CO_2$	minute carbon dioxide production
$\dot{V}O_2$	oxygen consumed
$\dot{V}CO_2/\dot{V}O_2$	respiratory exchange ratio
ΔXc	capacitive change in impedance
ΔZ	impedance change
Z	zone or impedance

8.0 REFERENCES

1. Utenick MR: Design of a hot wire anemometer. Biomed Sci Instrumen 7:46, 1970.

2. Godal A, Belenky DA, Standaert TA, et al.: Application of the hot wire anemometer to respiratory measurements in small animals. J Appl Physiol 40:275, 1976.

3. Baboolal R, Kirpalani H: Measuring on-line compliance in ventilated infants using hot wire anemometry. Crit Care Med 18:1070, 1990.

4. Demers RR, Saklad M: Respiratory mechanics. A theoretical and empirical approach. Respir Care 20:727–744, 1975.

5. Burton GG, Hodgkin JE: Respiratory Care. Philadelphia, J B Lippincott, 1984.

6. McPherson SP: Respiratory Therapy Equipment. Third Edition. St. Louis, C V Mosby Co., 1985.

7. Merläinen PT: A differential paramagnetic sensor for breath-by-breath oximetry. J Clin Monit 6:65–73, 1990.

8. Weingarten M: Respiratory monitoring of carbon dioxide and oxygen. A ten-year perspective. J Clin Monit 6:217–225, 1990.

9. Severinghäus JW, Astrup PB: History of blood gas analysis; IV Leland Clark's oxygen electrode. J Clin Monit 2:125–139, 1986.

10. Merläinen PT: Sensors for oxygen analysis: paramagnetic, electrochemical, polarographic, and zirconium oxide technologies. J Biomed Instrumen Technol 11/12:462–466, 1989.

11. Kocache R: The measurement of oxygen in gas mixtures. J Physiol E: Sci Instrumen 19:401–411, 1986.

12. Oxygen Monitors. ECRI Report. Product code 12-863, 1988.

13. Ilsley AH, Runciman WB: An evaluation of fourteen oxygen analyzers for use in patient breathing circuits. Anaesth Intens Care 14:431–6, 1986.

14. Krigman A: Moisture and humidity, 1985. An emphasis on sensor development. InTech 32:9–10, 1985.

15. Huang PH: Humidity sensing, measurements, and calibration standards. Sensors 12–21, 1990.

16. MacIntyre NR: Graphical Analysis of Flow, Pressure and Volume During Mechanical Ventilation. Third Edition. Riverside, Bear Medical Systems, Inc. 1991.

17. Waveforms: The Graphical Presentation of Ventilatory Data. Carlsbad, Puritan Bennett Corp, 1990.

18. Scheggi AM, Brenci M, Conforti G: Optical fibre thermometer for medical use. IEE Proceedings 131:270–272, 1984.

19. Tiny vane triggers optical pressure sensor. Machine Design 55:34, 1983.

20. Davis CM: Fiberoptic sensors; an overview. Optical Engineer 24:347–351, 1985.

21. Borman S: Optical and piezoelectric biosensors. Analyt Chem 59:1161–1162, 1987.

22. Flamang P, Sierens P: Study of the steady-state flow pattern in a multi-pulse converter by LDA (laser-doppler anemometry). J Engineer Gas Turb Power 110:515–522, 1988.

23. Linko K, Paloheimo M: Monitoring of the inspired and end-tidal oxygen, carbon dioxide, and nitrous oxide concentrations. Clinical applications during anesthesia and recovery. J Clin Monit 5:3, 1989.

24. Cole WG: Metaphor graphics and visual analogy for medical data. Delivered by William Cole at the Annual Symposium on Computer Applications in Medical Care, Washington D.C., 1987.

25. Cole WG: Quick and accurate monitoring via metaphor graphics, submitted to Symposium on Computer Applications in Medical Care (SCAMC), 1990.

26. Slutsky AS, Strohl KP: Quantification of oxygenation during episodicodic hypoxemia. Am Rev Respir Dir 121:893–895, 1980.

27. Squire JR: An instrument for measuring the quantity of blood and its degree of oxygenation in the web of the hand. Clin Sci 4:331–339, 1940.

28. Millikan GA: The oximeter, an instrument for measuring continuously the oxygen saturation of arterial blood in man. Rev Sci Instrumen 13:43–48, 1942.

29. Drabkin DL, Austin JH: A technique for the analysis of undiluted blood and concentrated hemoglobin solutions. J Biol Chem 112:1051–15, 1935.

30. Horecker BL: The absorption spectra of hemoglobin and its derivatives in the visible and near infrared regions. J Biol Chem 148:173–183, 1943.

31. Wood EH, Geraci JE: Photoelectric determination of arterial oxygen saturation in man. J Lab Clin Med 4:387–401, 1949.

32. Wukitsch MW, Patterson MT, Tonler DR, et al.: Pulse oximetry: Analysis of theory, technology, and practice. J Clin Monit 4:4 290–301, 1988.

33. Tremper KK, Barker SJ: Pulse oximetry. Anesthesiology 70:98–108, 1989.

34. Severinghäus JW, Naifeh KH: Accuracy of response of six pulse oximeters to profound hypoxia. Anesthesiology 67:551–558, 1987.

35. Penaz J: Photoelectric measurement of blood pressure, volume and flow in the finger. Digest 10th Intl Conf Med Biol Engineer 104, 1973.

36. Decker MJ, Dickensheets D, Arnold JL, et al.: A comparison of a new reflectance oximeter with the Hewlett Packard ear oximeter. Biomed Instrumen Technol 24:122–126, 1990.

37. Alexander CM, Teller LE, Gross JB: Principles of pulse oximetry: Theoretical and practical considerations. Anesth Analg 63:368–376, 1989.

38. Barker SJ, Tremper KK: The effect of carbon monoxide inhalation on pulse oximetry and transcutaneous PO_2. Anesthesiology 66:677–679, 1987.

39. Eisenkraft JB: Pulse oximeter desaturation due to the hemoglobinemia. Anesthesiology 68:2782–2792, 1988.

40. Kessler MR, Eide T, Humayun B, et al.: Spurious pulse oximeter desaturation with methylene blue injection. Anesthesiology 65:435–436, 1986.

41. Scheller MS, Unger RJ, Kelner MJ: Effects of intravenously administered dyes on pulse oximetry readings. Anesthesiology 65:550–552, 1986.

42. Brown DP, Cheung PW, Kenny MA, et al.: Theoretical models and experimental studies of pulse oximetry. IEEE Proceedings IX Congress, 435–441, 1987.

43. Cahan C, Decker MJ, Hoekje PL, et al.: Agreement between noninvasive oximetric values for oxygen saturation. Chest 97:814–819, 1990.

44. Strohl KP, House PM, Holic JF, et al.: Comparison of three transmittance oximeters. Med Instrumen 20:143–149, 1986.

45. Emergency Care Research Institute (ECRI): Health Devices, Pulse Oximeters. 18:208, 1989.

46. Amar D, Neidzwski J, Wald A, et al.: Fluorescent light interface with pulse oximetry. J Clin Monit 135–136, 1989.

47. Pologe JA: Pulse Oximetry: Technical aspects of machine design. In: International Anesthesiology Clinics: Advances in Oxygen Monitoring. Tremper KK, Barker SJ (Eds). Boston, Little Brown and Co., 1987.

48. Barker SJ, Tremper KK: Pulse oximetry: applications and limitations. In: International Anesthesiology Clinics: Advances in Oxygen Monitoring. Tremper KK, Barker SJ (Eds). Boston, Little Brown and Co., 1987.

49. Montenegro H, Decker MJ, Smith B, et al.: The effects of anemia and hypothermia on pulse oximetry monitoring in the I.C.U. Chest 88:118, 1990.

50. Palve H, Vuori A: Pulse oximetry during low cardiac output and hypothermia states immediately after open heart surgery. Crit Care Med 17:669, 1989.

51. Sloan T: Finger injury by an oxygen saturation monitor probe. Anesthesiology 68:936–938, 1988.

52. Schnapp LM, Cohen NH: Pulse oximetry, uses and abuses. Chest 98:1244–1250, 1990.

53. Merrill EW, Gilliland ER, Coklet G, et al.: Rheology of human blood near and at zero flow. Effects of temperature and hematocrit. Biophys J 3:199, 1963.

54. Berne RM, Levy MN (Eds): Physiology. St. Louis, CV Mosby Company, 1983.

55. Kramer K: Ein Verfahren zur fort laufenden messung des dauerstoffgehaltes im stronenden blute an uneroffneten getassen. Z Biol 96:61–75, 1935.

56. Matthes K, Gross F: Zur methode der fortlaufenden registrierung der farbe des menschlichen blutes. Arch Exp Pathol Pharmacol 191:523–528, 1939.

57. Millikan GA: The oximeter—an instrument for measuring continuously oxygen saturation of arterial blood in man. Rev Sci Instrumen 13:434–444, 1942.

58. Brinkman R, Ziljstra WG: Determination and continuous registration of the percentage oxygen saturation in small amounts of blood. Arch Chir Nerl 1:177–183, 1949.

59. Ware PF, Polanyi MC, Hehir RM, et al.: A new reflection oximeter. J Thorac Cardiovasc Surg 42:580–588, 1961.

60. Enson Y, Briscoe WA, Polanyi MC, et al.: In vivo studies with an intravascular and intracardiac reflection oximeter. J Appl Physiol 17:552–558, 1962.

61. Gettinger A, DeTraglia MC, Glass DD: In vivo comparison of two mixed venous catheters. Anesthesiology 66:372–375, 1987.

62. Rouby JJ, Poete P, Bodin L, et al.: Three mixed venous saturation catheters in patients with circulatory shock and respiratory failure. Chest 98:954–958, 1990.

63. Krasnitz P, Druger GL, Yorre F, et al.: Mixed venous oxygen tension and hyperlactemia: Survival in severe cardiopulmonary disease. JAMA 236:570–574, 1976.

64. Schweiss JF (Ed): Continuous Measurement of Blood Oxygen Saturtion in the High Risk Patient. San Diego, Beach International, Inc., 1983.

65. Jamieson WRE, Turnbull KW, Larrieu AJ, et al.: Continuous monitoring of mixed venous oxygen saturation in cardiac surgery. Can J Surg 25:538–542, 1982.

66. Krauss XH, Verdouw PD, Hugenholtz PG, et al.: On-line monitoring of mixed venous oxygen saturation after cardiothoracic surgery. Thorax 30:636–643, 1975.

67. Shoemaker WC, Appel P, Bland R: Use of physiologic monitoring to predict outcome and assist in clinical decisions in critically ill post-operative patients. Am J Surg 146:43–50, 1983.

68. Abraham E, Shoemaker WC, Bland RD, et al.: Sequential cardiorespiratory patterns in septic shock. Crit Care Med 11:799–803, 1983.

69. Nunn JF: Applied Respiratory Physiology. Third Edition. London, Butterworth & Co. Ltd., 1987.

70. Fahey PJ, Harris K, Van der Warf C: Clinical experience with continuous monitoring of mixed venous oxygen saturation in respiratory failure. Chest 86:748–752, 1984.

71. Laughlin TP, McMichan JC: Adjustment of PEEP according to continuous measurement of mixed venous O_2 saturation (SO_2) (Abst). Anesth Analg 63:242, 1984.

72. Morris AH, Chapman RH, Gardner RM: Frequency of technical problems encountered in the measurement of pulmonary-artery wedge pressure. Crit Care Med 12:164–170, 1984.

73. Johnston WE, Royster RL, Johansen VJ, et al.: Influence of balloon inflation and deflation on location of pulmonary artery catheter tip. Anesthesiology 67:110–115, 1987.

74. Orlando R: Continuous mixed venous oximetry in critically ill surgical patients: "high-tech" cost effectiveness. Arch Surg 121:4701, 1986.

75. Jastremski MS, Laksmipathi C, Beney KM, et al.: Analysis of the effects of continuous online monitoring of mixed venous oxygen saturation on patient outcome and cost effectiveness. Crit Care Med 17:148–152, 1989.

76. Forsyth RP, Hoffbrand BM, Melmon KL: Redistribution of cardiac output during hemorrhage in the unanesthetized monkey. Circ Res 27:311–320, 1970.

77. Astiz ME, Rackow EC, Falk JL, et al.: Oxygen delivery and consumption in patients with hypodynamic septic shock. Crit Care Med 15:26–28, 1987.

78. Vermeij CG, Bouke WA, Adrichem WJ, et al.: Dependent oxygen uptake and oxygen delivery in septic and post-operative patients. Chest 1438–1443, 1991.

79. Heiselman D, Jones J, Cannon L: Continuous monitoring of mixed venous oxygen saturation in septic shock. J Clin Monit 2:237–245, 1986.

80. Kyft JV, Vaughn S, Yang SC, et al.: Continuous monitoring of mixed venous oxygen saturation in patients with acute myocardial infarction. Chest 95:607–611, 1989.

81. Hasson E, Green JA, Nara AR, et al.: Continuous monitoring of mixed venous oxygen saturation as an indicator of pharmacologic intervention. Chest 95:406–409, 1989.

82. Jain A, Shroff SG, Janicki JS, et al.: Relation between mixed venous oxygen saturation and cardiac index: nonlinearity and normalization for oxygen uptake and hemoglobin. Chest 99:1403–1409, 1991.

83. Schlichting R, Cowden WL, Chaitman BR: Tolerance of unusually low mixed venous oxygen saturation: Adaptations in the chronic low cardiac output syndrome. Am J Med 813–818, 1986.

84. Fahey PJ (Ed): Continuous Measurement of Blood Oxygen Saturation in the High Risk Patient. Volume 2, San Diego, Beach International, Inc., 1985.

85. Barker SJ, Tremper KK, Hyatt J, et al.: Effects of methemoglobinemia on pulse oximetry and mixed venous oximetry (Abst). Anesthesiology 67:A170, 1987.

86. Rasanen J, Down JB, Malec DJ, et al.: Estimation of oxygen utilization by dual oximetry. Ann Surg 20:62–63, 1987.

87. Daily WJR, Klaus M, Meyer HBP: Apnea in premature infants; monitoring incidence, heart rate changes, and effect of environmental temperature. Pediatrics 45:510, 1969.

88. Stein IM, Shannon DC: The pediatric pneumogram: A new method for detecting and quantifying apnea in infants. Pediatrics 45:5–10, 1969.

89. Orr VC, Stahl ML, Duke H, et al.: Effect of sleep state and position on the incidence of obstruction and central apnea in infants. Pediatrics 75:832–850, 1985.

90. Nishino T, Hiraga K, Fujisato M, et al.: Breathing patterns during post-operative analgesia in patients after lower abdominal operations. Anesthesiology 69:967–972, 1988.

91. Consensus Development Statement On Infantile Apnea and Home Monitoring. In: Infantile Apnea and Home Monitoring (Report of Consensus Development Conference, September 29–October 1, 1986). Bethesda, Maryland, Department of Health and Human Services, 1987; NIH publication No. 87-2905. Section I:1–12.

92. Brouillette RT, Morrow AS, Weese-Mayer DE, et al.: Comparison of respiratory inductive plethysmography and thoracic impedance for apnea monitoring. J Pediatr 111:377–383, 1987.

93. Honma Y, Wilkes D, Bryan MH, et al.: Rib cage and abdominal contributions to ventilatory response to CO_2 in infants. J Appl Physiol 56(5):1211–1216, 1984.

94. Neuman MR: Apnea monitoring: technical aspects. Consensus Development Statement On Infantile Apnea and Home Monitoring. In: Infantile Apnea and Home Monitoring (Report of Consensus Development Conference, September 29–October 1, 1986). Bethesda, Maryland, Department of Health and Human Services; NIH publication No. 872–905, 1987.

95. Wright BM, Callan K: A new respiratory recording and monitoring system. In: Proceedings of the 3rd International Symposium on Ambulatory Monitoring, 1980. Stott FD, Raferty EB, Goulding L (Eds). London, Academic Press, 1980.

96. Guilleminault C, Ariagno R, Korobkin R, et al.: Sleep parameters and respiratory variables in "near miss" sudden infant death syndrome infants. Pediatrics 68:354–360, 1981.

97. Pacela AF: Impedance pneumography, a survey of instrumentation techniques. Med Biol Engineer 4:1–15, 1966.

98. Littwitz C, Ragheb T, Geddes LA: Cell constant of the tetrapolar conductivity cell. Med Biol Engineer Comput 28:587–590, 1990.

99. Yount JE: Easily calibrated circumferential respiratory effort transducer. Proceedings of the 11th International Conference IEEE and Engineering in Medicine and Biology, November, 1989.

100. Yount JE: Optimal detection sensitivity: a clinical perspective. In: Medical Technology for the Neonate. AAMI Technology Assessment report (TAR No. 9-8-4); Arlington, Virginia, Association for the Advancement of Medical Instrumentation, 1984.

101. Yount JE, Newcomb J, Hamill D, et al.: What method for accurate recognition of apnea? A blind quantitative study of thoracic impedance, abdominal pressure capsule, and abdominal circumference transducers. Am Rev Respir Dir 133:A367, 1986.

102. Yount JE, Benedetto W, Sherman P: Computerized multichannel database of respiratory waveforms to serve as model for monitor testing by ATS & FDA–Initial tests of current thoracic impedance and ECG monitors. Proceedings for ATS National Conference, May 1992, Am Rev Respir Dir, 1992.

103. Geddes LA, Foster KS, Reilly J, et al.: The rectification properties of an electrode-electrolyte interface operated at high sinusoidal current density. IEEE Trans Biomed Engineer BME 34:669–672, 1987.

104. AAMI Technical Information Report–Apnea monitoring by means of thoracic impedance pneumography. Arlington, Virginia, American Association for the Advancement of Medical Instrumentation, 1989.

105. Bouty, ME: Sur la conductibilite electrique des dissolutions salines tres etendues. J Physique 1884:3:325–355, 1984.

106. Schwan HP. Electrode polarization impedance and measurements in biological materials. Ann NY Acad Sci 148:191–209, 1986.

107. Yount JE, Neuman MR: Development of a physiologically appropriate circuit for testing thoracic impedance respiration monitors. Proceedings of XIV International Conference of Medical and Biological Engineering. Helsinki, Finland, August, 1985.

108. Salandin V, Zussa C, Risica G, et al.: Comparison of cardiac output estimation by thoracic electrical bio-impedance, thermodilution, and Fick methods. Crit Care Med 16:1157–1158, 1988.

109. Guardo R, Boulay C, Murray B, et al.: An experimental study in electrical impedance tomography. IEEE Trans Biomed Engineer BME- 38:617–627, 1991.

110. Shankar R, Webster JG: Noninvasive measurement of compliance of human leg arteries. IEEE Trans Bio-med Engineer BME-38:62–67, 1991.

111. Southall DP, Levitt GA, Richards JM, et al.: Undetected episodes of prolonged apnea and severe bradycardia in preterm infants. Pediatrics 72:541–542, 1983.

112. Phillipson EA, Bowes G: Control of breathing during sleep. In: Handbook of Physiology—The Respiratory System. Fishman AP, Cherniak NS, Widdicombe JG (Eds). Bethesda, Maryland, American Physiological Society, 1986.

113. Miller MJ, Waldemar AC, Martin RJ: Continuous positive airway pressure selectively reduces obstructive apnea in preterm infants. J Pediatr 106:91–94, 1985.

114. Lopes J, Muller NL, Bryan MH, Bryan AC: Importance of inspiratory muscle tone in maintenance of FRC in the newborn. J Appl Physiol 51:830–834, 1981.

115. Brouillette RT, Fernbach SK, Hunt CE: Obstructive sleep apnea in infants and children. J Pediatr 100:31–33, 1982.

116. Rigatto H, Desai U, Leahy F, et al.: The effect of 2% CO_2, 100% O_2, theophylline and 15% O_2 on "inspiratory drive" and "effective timing" in preterm infants. Early Hum Develop 5:63–70, 1981.

117. Cunningham DJC, Robbins PA, Wolff CB: Integration of respiratory responses to changes in alveolar partial pressures of CO_2 and O_2 and in arterial pH. In: Handbook of Physiology: The Respiratory System. Fishman AP, Cherniack NS, Widdicombe JG (Eds). Bethesda, Maryland, American Physiological Society, 1986.

118. Muller N, Gulston G, Cade D, et al.: Diaphragmatic muscle fatigue in the newborn. J Appl Physiol Resp Environ Exercise Physiol 46:688–695, 1979.

119. Druz WS, Sharp JT: Activity of respiratory muscles in upright and recumbent humans. J Appl Physiol 51:1552–1561, 1981.

120. Staats BA, Bonekat HW, Harris CD, et al.: Chest wall motion in sleep apnea. Am Rev Respir Dir 130:59–63, 1984.

121. AAMI Apnea Monitor Standards Committee Minutes of Meeting, November 25, 1991. Arlington, Virginia, Association for the Advancement of Medical Instrumentation, 1991.

122. Richards JM, Alexander JR, Shinebourne EA, et al.: Sequential 22-hour profiles of breathing patterns and heart rate in 110 full-term infants during their first 6 months of life. Pediatrics 74:763–777, 1984.

123. Welborn LG, Hannallah RS, Fink R, et al.: High dose caffeine suppresses postoperative apnea in former preterm infants. Anesthesiology 71:347–349, 1989.

124. Martin RJ, Miller MJ, Carlo WA: Pathogenesis of apnea in preterm infants. J Pediatr 109:733–741, 1986.

125. Marchal F, Bairam A, Vert P: Neonatal apnea and apneic syndromes. In: The respiratory system in the newborn. Clin Perinatal 14:509–529, 1987.

126. Oren J, Kelly D, Shannon DC: Identification of a high-risk group for sudden infant death syndrome among infants who were resuscitated for sleep apnea. Pediatrics 77:495–499, 1986.

127. Apnea. In: Infantile Apnea and Home Monitoring (Report of Consensus Development Conference, September 29–October 1, 1986). Bethesda, Maryland, Department of Health and Human Services, NIH publication No. 87-2905. Section II 2:1–25 and Appendix B:23–51, 1987.

128. Booth CL, Morin VN, Waite SP, et al.: Periodic and nonperiodic sleep apnea in premature and full-term infants. Dev Med Child Neurol 25:283–296, 1983.

129. Khoo MC, Kronauer RE, Strohl KP, et al.: Factors inducing periodic breathing in humans: A general model. J Appl Physiol 53:644–659, 1982.

130. Weil JV: Ventilatory control at high altitude. In: Handbook of Physiology: The Respiratory System. Fishman AP, Cherniack NS, Widdicombe JG (Eds). Bethesda, Maryland, American Physiological Society, 1986.

131. Purves MJ: Fluctuations of arterial oxygen tension which have the same period as respiration. Respir Physiol 1:1281–1296, 1966.

132. Guilleminault C, McQuitty J, Ariagno RL, et al.: Congenital central alveolar hypoventilation syndrome in six infants. Pediatrics 70:684–694, 1982.

133. Roussos C, MacKlen PT: Inspiratory muscle fatigue. In: Handbook of Physiology–The Respiratory System. Fishman AP, Cherniak NS, Widdicombe JG (Eds). Bethesda, Maryland, American Physiological Society, 1986.

134. Paton JY, Swaminathan S, Sargent CW, et al.: Hypoxic and hypercapnic ventilatory responses in awake children with congenital central hypoventilation syndrome. Am Rev Respir Dir 140:368–372, 1989.

135. Oren J, Kelly DH, Shannon DC: Long-term follow-up of children with congenital central hypoventilation syndrome. Pediatrics 80:375–380, 1987.

136. Ross RD, Daniels SR, Loggie JMH, et al.: Sleep apnea associated hypertension and reversible left ventricular hypertrophy. J Pediatr 111:253–255, 1987.

137. Ward SLD, Nickerson BG, van der Hal A, et al.: Absent hypoxic and hypercapneic arousal responses in children with myelomeningocele and apnea. Pediatrics 78:44–50, 1986.

138. Neuman MR: Apnea monitoring: technical aspects. In Consensus Development Statement on Infantile Apnea and Home Monitoring. In: Infantile Apnea and Home Monitoring (Report of Consensus Development Conference, September 29–October 1, 1986). Bethesda, Maryland, Department of Health and Human Services, NIH publication No. 87-2905, 1987.

139. Yount JE, Neuman MR: Development of a physiologically appropriate circuit for testing thoracic impedance respiration monitors. Proceedings of XIV International Conference of Medical and Biological Engineering, Helsinki, Finland, August, 1985.

9.0 ILLUSTRATION CREDITS

Figure 1.2
Levitzky MG, Cairo JM, Hall SM: Introduction to Respiratory Care. Philadelphia, WB Saunders, 1990.

Figure 1.3
Murray JS: The Normal Lung. Second Edition. Philadephia, WB Saunders, 1986.

Figure 1.4
Fishman AP: Pulmonary Diseases and Disorders. Second Edition. Vol. 1, New York, McGraw-Hill Book Company, 1988.

Figure 1.5
Hammond EC: The effects of smoking. New York, Scientific American, Inc., 1962.

Figure 1.6
Shapiro B, Harrison R, Trout C: Clinical Applications of Respiratory Care. Second Edition. Chicago, Year Book Medical Publishers, 1979.

Figure 1.8
Shapiro B, Harrison R, Trout C: Clinical Applications of Respiratory Care. Second Edition. Chicago, Year Book Medical Publishers, 1979.

Figure 1.9
West JB: Respiratory Physiology—The Essentials. Baltimore, Williams and Wilkins Company, 1974.

Figure 1.10
West JB: Ventilation—Blood Flow and Gas Exchange. Cambridge, Blackwell Scientific Publications, 1977.

Figure 1.12
Shapiro B, Harrison R, Trout C: Clinical Applications of Respiratory Care. Second Edition. Chicago, Year Book Medical Publishers, 1979.

Figure 1.13
West JB: Ventilation—Blood Flow and Gas Exchange. Fourth Edition. Cambridge, Blackwell Scientific Publications, 1985.

Figure 1.15
Shapiro B, Harrison R, Walton J: Clinical Applications of Blood Gases. Third Edition. Chicago, Year Book Medical Publishers, 1982.

Figure 1.16
Scanlan CL, Spearman EB, Sheldon RL: Egan's Fundamentals of Respiratory Care. St. Louis, CV Mosby Company, 1990.

Figure 1.17
Mines AH: Respiratory Physiology. Second Edition. New York, Raven Press, 1986.

Figure 1.18
Levitzky MG: Pulmonary Physiology. Second Edition. New York, McGraw-Hill, 1986.

Figure 1.19
West JB: Ventilation—Blood Flow and Gas Exchange. Fourth Edition. Cambridge, Blackwell Scientific Publications, 1985.

Figure 1.20
Shapiro B, Harrison R, Trout C: Clinical Applications of Respiratory Care. Second Edition. Chicago, Year Book Medical Publishers, 1979.

Figure 1.21
West JB: Ventilation—Blood Flow and Gas Exchange. Fourth Edition. Cambridge, Blackwell Scientific Publications, 1985.

Figure 1.22
West JB: Respiratory Physiology—The Essentials. Baltimore, Williams and Wilkins Company, 1974.

Figure 1.23
West JB: Ventilation—Blood Flow and Gas Exchange. Fourth Edition. Cambridge, Blackwell Scientific Publications, 1985.

Figure 1.24
Shapiro B, Harrison R, Walton J: Clinical Application of Blood Gases. Third Edition. Chicago, Year Book Medical Publishers, 1982.

Figure 1.25
McLaughlin A: Essentials of Physiology for Advanced Respiratory Therapy. St. Louis, CV Mosby Company, 1977.

Figure 1.30
West JB: Respiratory Physiology—The Essentials. Baltimore, Williams and Wilkins Company, 1974.

Figure 3.2
Wukitsch M: Pulse oximetry: analysis of theory, technology and practice. Boston, J Clin Monit 4:291, 1988.

Figure 3.4
Wukitsch M: Pulse oximetry: analysis of theory, technology and practice. Boston, J Clin Monit 4:294, 1988.

Figure 3.5
Wukitsch M: Pulse oximetry: analysis of theory, technology and practice. J Clin Monit 4:293, 1988.

Figure 3.6
Wukitsch M: Pulse oximetry: analysis of theory, technology and practice. J Clin Monit 4:292, 1988.

Figure 4.1
Reinhart K: Principles and Practice of SO_2 Monitoring. Intensive Care World 5:122, 1988.

Figure 4.2
Miller JD, Cucchiara B (Eds): Anesthesia. Second Edition. New York, Churchill Livingstone, 1986.

Figure 4.3
Fahey PJ (Ed): Continuous Measurement of Blood Oxygen Saturation in the High Risk Patient. San Diego, Beach International, Inc., 1985.

Figure 4.4
Fahey PJ (Ed): Continuous Measurement of Blood Oxygen Saturation in the High Risk Patient. San Diego, Beach International, Inc., 1985.

Figure 4.5
Fahey PJ (Ed): Continuous Measurement of Blood Oxygen Saturation in the High Risk Patient. San Diego, Beach International, Inc., 1985.

Figure 4.6
Fahey PJ (Ed): Continuous Measurement of Blood Oxygen Saturation in the High Risk Patient. San Diego, Beach International, Inc., 1985.

Figure 4.7
Gravenstein JS, Paulus DA: Clinical Monitoring Practice. Philadelphia, JB Lippincott Company, 1987.

Figure 4.8
Gravenstein JS, Paulus DA: Clinical Monitoring Practice. Philadelphia, JB Lippincott Company, 1987.

Figure 4.9
Nunn JF: Applied Respiratory Physiology. London, Butterworth & Company, Ltd., 1987.

Figure 5.2
Druz WS, Sharp JT: Activity of respiratory muscles in upright and recumbent humans. J Appl Physiol Respir Environ Exercise Physiol 51:1552–1561, 1981.

Figure 5.3
Honma Y, Wilkes D, Bryan MH: Rib cage and abdominal contributions to ventilatory response to CO_2 in infants. J Appl Physiol Respir Environ Exercise Physiol 56:1211–1216, 1984.

Figure 5.6
Lopes J, Muller NL, Bryan MH, et al.: Importance of inspiratory muscle tone in maintenance of FRC the newborn. J Appl Physiol Respir Environ Exercise Pysiol 51:830–834, 1981.

Figure 6.2
Gravenstein JS, Paulus DA, Hayes TJ: Capnography in Clinical Practice. Boston, Butterworths, 1989.

Figure 6.3
Fletcher R, Werner O, Nordstrom L, et al.: Sources of error and their correction in the measurement of carbon dioxide elimination using the Siemens-Elema CO_2 analyzer. Br J Anaesth 55:177, 1983.

Figure 6.4
Adapted from Gravenstein JS, Paulus DA, Hayes TJ: Capnography in Clinical Practice. Boston, Butterworths, 1989.

Figure 6.5
Kleiger R, Miller J, Bigger J, et al.: Decreased heart rate variability and its association with increased mortality after acute myocardial infarction. Am J Cardiol 59:256, 1987.

Figure 6.6 (b)
Adapted from Szaflarski NJ, Cohen NH: Use of capnography in critically ill adults. Heart Lung 20:363, 1991.

Figure 6.13
Salter Labs, Arvin, California, Salter Divided Cannulae brochure, 1991.

10.0 BIBLIOGRAPHY

The following bibliography lists, in chronological order, citations pertinent to the study of respiration.

10.1 Pulmonary Physiology

Hammond EC: The effects of smoking. New York, Scientific American, Inc., 1962.

West JB: Respiratory Physiology—The Essentials. Baltimore, Williams and Wilkins Company, 1974.

McLaughlin A: Essentials of Physiology for Advanced Respiratory Therapy. St. Louis, CV Mosby Company, 1977.

West JB: Ventilation—Blood Flow and Gas Exchange. Cambridge, Blackwell Scientific Publications, 1977.

Shapiro B, Harrison R, Trout C: Clinical Applications of Respiratory Care. Second Edition. Chicago, Year Book Medical Publishers, 1979.

Shapiro B, Harrison R, Walton J: Clinical Application of Blood Gases. Third Edition. Chicago, Year Book Medical Publishers, 1982.

West JB: Ventilation—Blood Flow and Gas Exchange. Fourth Edition. Cambridge, Blackwell Scientific Publications, 1985.

Mines AH: Respiratory Physiology. Second Edition. New York, Raven Press, 1986.

Levitzky MG: Pulmonary Physiology. Second Edition. New York, McGraw-Hill Book Company, 1986.

Murray JS: The Normal Lung. Second Edition. Philadelphia, WB Saunders Company, 1986.

Fishman AP: Pulmonary Diseases and Disorders. Second Edition. Vol. 1. New York, McGraw-Hill Book Company, 1988.

Scanlan CL, Spearman CB, Sheldon RL: Egan's Fundamentals of Respiratory Care. St. Louis, CV Mosby Company, 1990.

Levitzky MG, Cairo JM, Hall SM: Introduction to Respiratory Care. Philadelphia, WB Saunders, 1990.

10.2 Airway Monitoring of the Adult, Pediatric, and Neonatal Patients

Utenick MR: Design of a hot wire anemometer. Biomed Sci Instrumen 7:46, 1970.

Demers RR, Saklad M: Respiratory mechanics; A theoretical and empirical approach. Respir Care 20:727–744, 1975.

Godal A, Belenky DA, Standaert TA, et al.: Application of the hot wire anemometer to respiratory measurements in small animals. J Appl Physiol 40:275, 1976.

Tiny vane triggers optical pressure sensor. Machine Design 55:34, 1983.

Burton GG, Hodgkin JE: Respiratory Care. Philadelphia, JB Lippincott, 1984.

Scheggi AM, Brenci M, Conforti G: Optical fibre thermometer for medical use. IEE Proceedings 131: 270–272, 1984.

Davis CM: Fiberoptic sensors: an overview. Optical Engineer 24: 347–351, 1985.

McPherson SP: Respiratory Therapy Equipment. Third Edition. St. Louis, CV Mosby Co., 1985.

Krigman A: Moisture and humidity. An emphasis on sensor development. InTech 32:9–10, 1985.

Severinghaus JW, Astrup PB: History of blood gas analysis; IV Leland Clark's oxygen electrode. J Clin Monit 2:125–139, 1986.

Kocache R: The measurement of oxygen in gas mixtures. J Physiol E: Sci Instrumen 19:401–411, 1986.

Ilsley AH, Runciman WB: An evaluation of fourteen oxygen analyzers for use in patient breathing circuits. Anaesthesiol Intens Care 14:431–436, 1986.

Oxygen Monitors. ECRI Report. Product code 12-863, October 1988.

Cole WG: Metaphor graphics and visual analogy for medical data. Delivered by William Cole at the Annual Symposium on Computer Applications in Medical Care, Washington D.C., October 1987.

Borman S: Optical and piezoelectric biosensors. Analyt Chem 59:1161–1162, 1987.

Flamang P, Sierens P: Study of the steady-state flow pattern in a multipulse converter by LDA (Laser-Doppler Anemometry). J Engineer Gas Turb Power 110:515–522, 1988.

Linko K, Paloheimo M: Monitoring of the inspired and end-tidal oxygen, carbon dioxide, and nitrous oxide concentrations; Clinical applications during anesthesia and recovery. J Clin Monit 5:3, 1989.

Merläinen PT: Sensors for oxygen analysis: ara-magnetic, electrochemical, polarographic, and zirconium oxide technologies. J Biomed Instrumen Tech 11/12:462–466, 1989.

Baboolal R, Kirpalani H: Measuring on-line compliance in ventilated infants using hot wire anemometry. Crit Care Med 18:1070, 1990.

Merläinen PT: A differential paramagnetic sensor for breath-by-breath oximetry. J Clin Monit 6:65–73, 1990.

Weingarten M: Respiratory monitoring of carbon dioxide and oxygen; A ten-year perspective. J Clin Monit 6:217–225, 1990.

Cole WG: Quick and accurate monitoring via metaphor graphics, submitted to Symposium on Computer Applications in Medical Care (SCAMC), 1990.

Huang PH: Humidity sensing, measurements, and calibration standards. Sensors 12–21, 1990.

Waveforms: The Graphical Presentation of Ventilatory Data. Carlsbad, Puritan Bennett Corp., 1990.

MacIntyre NR: Graphical Analysis of Flow, Pressure and Volume During Mechanical Ventilation, Third Edition. Riverside, Bear Medical Systems, Inc., 1991.

10.3 Pulse Oximetry

Loewinger E, Gordon A, Winreb A, et al.: Analysis of a micromethod for transmission oximetry of whole blood. J Appl Physiol 19:1179–1184, 1964.

Mook GA, van Assendelft OW, Zijlstra WG: Wavelength dependency of the spectrophotometric determination of blood oxygen saturation. Clin Chem Acta 26:170–173, 1969.

Nakajimi S, Hirai S, Takase H, et al.: New pulsed-type earpiece oximeter (English translation). Kokyu To Junkan 23:709–713, 1975.

Saunders NA, Powles AC, Rebuck AS: Ear oximetry practicability in the assessment of arterial oxygenation. Am Rev Respir Dir 113:745–749, 1976.

Asari M, Kenmotsu O: Application of a pulse-type earpiece oximeter in the field of anesthesiology. Masui 26:205–208, 1977.

Douglas NJ, Brash HK, Wraith PK, et al.: Accuracy sensitivity to carboxyhemoglobin, and speed of response to the Hewlett-Packard 47201A ear oximeter. Am Rev Respir Dir 119:311–313, 1979.

Stradling JR: The accuracy of the Hewlett-Packard 47201A ear oximeter below 50% saturation. Bull Eur Physiopathol Respir 18:791–794, 1982.

Chapman KR, D'Urzo A, Rebuck AS: The accuracy and response characteristics of a simplified ear oximeter. Chest 83:860–864, 1983.

Brooks TD, Paulus DA, Winkle WE: Infrared heat lamps interfere with pulse oximeters (letter). Anesthesiology 61:630, 1984.

Kim JM, Mathewson HS: Venous congestion affects arterial hemoglobin saturation measured by the pulse oximeter. Anesthesiology 63:A174, 1985.

Chapman KR, Liu FR, Watson RM, et al.: Range of accuracy of two-wavelength oximetry. Chest 89:540–542, 1986.

Kim JM, Arakawa K, Benson KT, et al.: Pulse oximetry and circulatory kinetics associated with pulse volume amplitude measured by photo-electric plethysmography. Anesth Analg 65:1333–1339, 1986.

Payne JP, Severinhause JW (Eds): Pulse Oximetry. Great Britain, Springer-Werlag Berlin Heidelberg, 1986.

Sidi A, Paulus DA, Rush W, et al.: Methylene blue and indocyanine green artifactually lower pulse oximetry readings of oxygen saturation. Studies in dogs. J Clin Monit 3:249–256, 1987.

Costarino AT, Davis DA, Leon TP: Falsely normal saturation reading with the pulse oximeter. Anesthesiology 67:830–831, 1987.

Block FE: Interference in a pulse oximeter from a fiberoptic light source. J Clin Monit 3:210–211, 1987.

Lawson D, Norley I, Korbon G, et al.: Blood flow limits and pulse oximeter signal detection. Anesthesiology 67:599–603, 1987.

Severinghaus JW: History status and future of pulse oximetry. Anesthesiology 67:864–865, 1987.

Neumann MR: Pulse oximetry, physical principles, technical realization and present limitations. Adv Exp Med Biol 220:135–144, 1987.

Nickerson BG, Sarkisan C, Tremper K: Bias and precision of pulse oximeters and arterial oximeters. Chest 93:515–517, 1988.

Decker MJ, Hoekje PL, Strohl KP: Ambulatory monitoring of arterial oxygen saturation. Chest 95:717–722, 1989.

10.4 Mixed Venous Oxygen

Rodrigo FA: The determination of the oxygenation of blood in vitro by using reflected light. Am Heart J 45:809–822, 1953.

Swan HJC, Ganz W, Forrester J, et al.: Catheterization of the heart in man with use of a flow-directed balloon-type catheter. N Eng J Med 283:447–451, 1970.

Cole JS, Martin WE, Cheung PW, et al.: Clinical studies with a solid state fiberoptic oximeter. Am J Cardiol 29:383–388, 1972.

Finch CA, Lenfant C: Oxygen transport in man. N Engl J Med 286:407–410, 1972.

Taylor JB, Lown B, Polanyi M: In vivo monitoring with a fiberoptic catheter. JAMA 221:667–673, 1972.

Wilkinson AR, Phibbs RH, Gregory GA: Continuous measurement of oxygen saturation in sick newborn infants. J Pediat 93:1016–1019, 1978.

De La Rocha AG, Edmonds JF, Williams WG, et al.: Importance of mixed venous oxygen saturation in the care of critically ill patients. Can J Surg 21:227–229, 1978.

Hechtman HB, Grindlinger GA, Vegas AM, et al.: Importance of oxygen transport in clinical medicine. Crit Care Med 7:419–429, 1979.

Birman J, Hew E, Aberman A: Continuous monitoring of mixed venous oxygen saturation in hemodynamically unstable patients. Chest 86:753–756, 1984.

Gore JM, Sloan K: Use of continuous monitoring of mixed venous oxygen saturation in the coronary care unit. Chest 86:757–761, 1984.

Rah KH, Dunwiddie WC, Lower RR: A method for continuous postoperative measurement of mixed venous oxygen saturation in infants and children after open heart procedures. Anesth Analg 63:873–881, 1984.

Harris K: New respiratory critical care technologies: Will they survive under prospective reimbursement? AART Times 8:35–39, 1984.

Bland RD, Shoemaker WC: Common physiologic patterns in general surgical patients: Hemodynamic and oxygen transport changes during and after operation in patients with and without associated medical problems. Surg Clin N Am 65:793–809, 1985.

Brown EG, Krouskop RW, McDonnell FE, et al.: A technique to continuously measure arteriovenous oxygen content difference and P_{50} in vivo. J Appl Physiol 58:1383–1389, 1985.

Norfleet E, Watson C: Continuous mixed venous oxygen saturation measurement: A significant advance in hemodynamic monitoring? J Clin Monit 1:245–256, 1985.

Severinghaus JW, Astrup PB: History of blood gas analysis. VI. Oximetry. J Clin Monit 2:270–288, 1986.

Davies G, Jebson PJR, Glasgow BM, et al.: continuous Fick cardiac output compared to thermodilution cardiac output. Crit Care Med 14:881–885, 1986.

Boutros AR, Lee C: Value of monitoring of mixed venous blood oxygen saturation in the management of critically ill patients. Crit Care Med 14:132–134, 1986.

Buran MJ: Oxygen Consumption. In: Oxygen Transport in the Critically Ill. Snyder JV, Pinsky MR (Eds). Chicago, Year Book Medical Publishers, 1987.

Gettinger A, DeTraglia MC, Glass DD: In vivo comparison of two mixed venous saturation catheters. Anesthiology 66:373–375, 1987.

Kirshon DB, Cotton DB: Invasive hemodynamic monitoring in the obstetric patient. Clin Obstet Gynecol 30:579–590, 1987.

Nelson LD: Venous Oximetry. In: Oxygen Transport in the Critically Ill Patient. Snyder JV (Ed). Chicago, Year Book Medical Publishers, 1987.

Gelman S, McDowell H, Vamer PD, et al.: The reason for cardiac output reduction after aortic cross-clamping. Am J Surg 155:578–785, 1988.

Thys DM, Cohen E, Eisenkraft JB: Mixed venous oxygen saturation during thoracic anesthesia. Anesthesiology 69:1005–1009, 1988.

Vaughn S, Puri VK: Cardiac output changes and continuous mixed venous oxygen saturation measurement in the critically ill. Crit Care Med 16:495–498, 1988.

Reinhard K: Principles and practice of SO_2 monitoring. Intens Care World 5:121–124, 1988.

Kupeli IA, Satwicz PR: Mixed venous oximetry. Intern Anesthesiol Clin 27:176–183, 1989.

Rasanen J, Downs JB, Hodges MR: Continuous monitoring of gas exchange and oxygen use with dual oximetry. J Clin Anesthesiol 1:3–8, 1988.

Varon AJ, Anderson HB, Civetta JM: Desaturation noted by pulmonary artery catheter after methylene blue injection. Anesthesiology 71:792–794, 1989.

Rafkin HS, Crippen DW, Hoyt JW: Dual oximetry as a real time monitor of cardiac function (Abst). Chest 96:289S, 1989.

Civetta JM: Simultaneous arterial and venous oximetry. Crit Care Updates 1:1–12, 1990.

Benumof JL: Respiratory Physiology and Respiratory Function During Anesthesia. In: Anesthesia, Third Edition. Miller RD, Cucchiara RF, Miller ED, et al. (Eds). New York, Churchill Livingstone, 1990.

Howdieshall T, Sussman A, Dipiro J, et al.: The reliability of mixed venous oximetry during intralipid infusion (Abst). Crit Care Med 18:S185, 1990.

Van Riper DF, Horrow JC, Kutalek SP, et al.: Mixed venous oximetry during automatic implantable cardioverter defibrillator placement. Transport 1:3–7, 1990.

Tremper KK, Barker SJ: Monitoring of Oxygen, In: Clinical Monitoring. Lake CL (Ed). Philadelphia, WB Saunders, 1990.

White KM: The effects of routine nursing care on the oxygen supply/demand balance of critically ill patients. Transport 2:5–10, 1991.

10.5 Impedence Pneumography

Pacela AF: Impedance pneumography, a survey of instrumentation techniques. Med Biol Engineer 4:1–15, 1966.

Purves MJ: Fluctuations of arterial oxygen tension which have the same period as respiration. Respir Physiol :1281–1296, 1966.

Daily WJR, Klaus M, Meyer HBP: Apnea in premature infants; monitoring incidence, heart rate changes, and effect of environmental temperature. Pediatrics 45:510, 1969.

Stein IM, Shannon DC: The pediatric pneumogram: A new method for detecting and quantifying apnea in infants. Pediatrics 45:510, 1969.

Muller N, Gulston G, Cade D, et al.: Diaphragmatic muscle fatigue in the newborn. J Appl Physiol: Respir Environ Exercise Physiol 46:688–695, 1979.

Wright BM, Callan K: A new respiratory recording and monitoring system. In: Proceedings of the 3rd International Symposium on Ambulatory Monitoring, 1980. Stott FD, Raferty EB, Goulding L (Eds). London, Academic Press, 1980.

Lopes J, Muller NL, Bryan MH, et al.: Importance of inspiratory muscle tone in maintenance of FRC in the newborn. J Appl Physiol 51:830–834, 1981.

Guilleminault C, Ariagno R, Korobkin R, et al.: Sleep parameters and respiratory variables in "near miss" sudden infant death syndrome infants. Pediatrics 68:354–360, 1981.

Rigatto H, Desai U, Leahy F, et al.: The effect of 2% CO_2, 100% O_2, theophylline and 15% O_2 on "inspiratory drive" and "effective timing" in preterm infants. Early Hum Develop 5:63–70, 1981.

Druz WS, Sharp JT: Activity of respiratory muscles in upright and recumbent humans. J Appl Physiol 51:1552–1561, 1981.

Brouillette RT, Fernbach SK, Hunt CE: Obstructive sleep apnea in infants and children. J Pediatr 100:31, 1982.

Guilleminault C, McQuitty J, Ariagno RL, et al.: Congenital central alveolar hypoventilation syndrome in six infants. Pediatrics 70:684–694, 1982.

Khoo MC, Kronauer RE, Strohl KP, et al.: Factors inducing periodic breathing in humans: a general model. J Appl Physiol 53:644–659, 1982.

Southall DP, Levitt GA, Richards JM, et al.: Undetected episodes of prolonged apnea and severe bradycardia in preterm infants. Pediatrics 72:541, 1983.

Booth CL, Morin VN, Waite SP, et al.: Periodic and nonperiodic sleep apnea in premature and full-term infants. Develop Med Child Neurol 25:283–296, 1983.

Staats BA, Bonekat HW, Harris CD, et al.: Chest wall motion in sleep apnea. Am Rev Respir Dir 130:59–63, 1984.

Honma Y, Wilkes D, Bryan MH, et al.: Rib cage and abdominal contributions to ventilatory response to CO_2 in infants. J Appl Physiol 56:1211–1216, 1984.

Richards JM, Alexander JR, Shinebourne EA, et al.: Sequential 22-hour profiles of breathing patterns and heart rate in 110 full-term infants during their first 6 months of life. Pediatrics 74:763–777, 1984.

Yount JE, Optimal detection sensitivity: a clinical perspective. In: Medical Technology for the Neonate. AAMI Technology Assessment report (TAR No. 9-84); Arlington, Virginia, Association for the Advancement of Medical Instrumentation, 1984.

Bouty, ME: Sur la conductibilite electrique des dissolutions salines tres etendues. J Physique 1884:325–355, 1984.

Orr VC, Stahl ML, Duke H, et al.: Effect of sleep state and position on the incidence of obstruction and central apnea in infants. Pediatrics 75:832–850, 1985.

Yount JE, Neuman MR: Development of a physiologically appropriate circuit for testing thoracic impedance respiration monitors. Proceedings of XIV International Conference of Medical and Biological Engineering. Helsinki, Finland, August, 1985.

Miller MJ, Waldemar AC, Martin RJ: Continuous positive airway pressure selectively reduces obstructive apnea in preterm infants. J Pediatr 106:91–94, 1985.

Schwan HP: Electrode polarization impedance and measurements in biological materials. Ann NY Acad Sci 148:191–209, 1986.

Yount JE, Newcomb J, Hamill D, et al.: What method for accurate recognition of apnea? A blind quantitative study of thoracic impedance, abdominal pressure capsule, and abdominal circumference transducers. Am Rev Respir Dir 133:A367, 1986.

Ward SLD, Nickerson BG, van der Hal A, et al.: Absent hypoxic and hypercapnic arousal responses in children with myelomeningocele and apnea. Pediat 78:44–50, 1986.

Weil JV: Ventilatory control at high altitude. In: Handbook of Physiology: The Respiratory System. Fishman AP, Cherniack NS, Widdicombe JG (Eds). Bethesda, Maryland, American Physiological Society, 1986.

Oren J, Kelly D, Shannon DC: Identification of a high-risk group for sudden infant death syndrome among infants who were resuscitated for sleep apnea. Pediatrics 77:495–499, 1986.

Martin RJ, Miller MJ, Carlo WA: Pathogenesis of apnea in preterm infants. J Pediatr 109:733–741, 1986.

Consensus Development Statement On Infantile Apnea and Home Monitoring. In: Infantile Apnea and Home Monitoring (Report of Consensus Development Conference, September 29–October 1, 1986). Bethesda, Maryland, Department of Health and Human Services, 1987; NIH publication No. 87-2905. Section I:1–12.

Brouillette RT, Morrow AS, Weese-Mayer DE, et al.: Comparison of respiratory inductive plethysmography and thoracic impedance for apnea monitoring. J Pediatr 111:377–383, 1987.

Geddes LA, Foster KS, Reilly J, et al.: The rectification properties of an electrode-electrolyte interface operated at high sinusoidal current density. IEEE Trans Biomed Engineer BME-34:669–672, 1987.

Oren J, Kelly DH, Shannon DC: Long-term follow-up of children with congenital central hypoventilation syndrome. Pediatrics 80:375–380, 1987.

Ross RD, Daniels SR, Loggie JMH, et al.: Sleep apnea-associated hypertension and reversible left ventricular hypertrophy. J Pediatr 111:253–225, 1987.

Marchal F, Bairam A, Vert P: Neonatal apnea and apneic syndromes. In: The respiratory system in the newborn. Clin Perinatal 14:509–529, 1987.

Salandin V, Zussa C, Risica G, et al.: Comparison of cardiac output estimation by thoracic electrical bioimpedance, thermodilution, and Fick methods. Crit Care Med 16:1157–1158, 1988.

Neuman MR: Apnea monitoring: Technical aspects. Consensus Development Statement On Infantile Apnea and Home Monitoring. In: Infantile Apnea and Home Monitoring (Report of Consensus Development Conference, September 29–October 1, 1986). Bethesda, Maryland, Department of Health and Human Services, 1987.

Nishino T, Hiraga K, Fujisato M, et al.: Breathing patterns during postoperative analgesia in patients after lower abdominal operations. Anesthesiology 69:967–972, 1988.

Yount JE: Easily calibrated circumferential respiratory effort transducer. Proceedings of the 11th International Conference IEEE and Engineering in Medicine and Biology, November 1989.

Welborn LG, Hannallah RS, Fink R, et al.: High dose caffeine suppresses postoperative apnea in former preterm infants. Anesthesiology 71:347–349, 1989.

AAMI Technical Information Report—Apnea monitoring by means of thoracic impedance pneumography. Arlington, Virginia, American Association for the Advancement of Medical Instrumentation, 1989.

Paton JY, Swaminathan S, Sargent CW, et al.: Hypoxic and hypercapnic ventilatory responses in awake children with congenital central hypoventilation syndrome. Am Rev Respir Dir 140:368–372, 1989.

Littwitz C, Ragheb T, Geddes LA: Cell constant of the tetrapolar conductivity cell. Med Biol Engineer Comput 28:587–590, 1990.

AAMI Apnea Monitor Standards Committee Minutes of Meeting, November 25, 1991. Arlington, Virginia, Association for the Advancement of Medical Instrumentation, 1991.

Guardo R, Boulay C, Murray B, et al.: An experimental study in electrical impedance tomography. IEEE Trans Biomed Engineer BME-38:617–627, 1991.

Shankar R, Webster JG: Noninvasive measurement of compliance of human leg arteries. IEEE Trans Biomed Engineer BME-38:62–67, 1991.

Yount JE, Benedetto W, Sherman P: Computerized multichannel database of respiratory waveforms to serve as model for monitor testing by ATS & FDA—initial tests of current thoracic impedance and ECG monitors. Proceedings for ATS—National Conference May 1992, Am Rev Respir Dir, 1992.

10.6 Capnography and Gas Monitoring

Rahn H, Farhi LE: Ventilation, Perfusion, and Gas Exchange—the V_A/Q Concept. In: Handbook of Physiology, Section 3 Respiration, Vol. 1. Fenn WO, Rahn H (Eds). Washington DC, American Physiology Society, 1954.

Rossier PH, Buhlmann AA, Weisinger K: Respiration; Physiological Principles and Their Clinical Applications. St. Louis, CV Mosby, 1960.

Hoffbrand BI: The expiratory capnogram; a measure of ventilation-perfusion inequalities. Thorax 21:518–523, 1966.

Kuwabara S, Duncalf D: Effect of anatomic shunt on physiologic deadspace-to-tidal volume ratio; a new equation. Anesthesiology 31:575–577, 1969.

Smalhout B, Kalenda A: An Atlas of Capnography. The Netherlands, Kerkebosch-Zeist, 1975.

Luft UC, Loepsky JA, Mostyn EM: Mean alveolar gases and alveolar-arterial gradients in pulmonary patients. J Appl Physiol 46:534–540, 1979.

Burki NK, Albert RK: Noninvasive monitoring of arterial blood gases: A report of the ACCP section on respiratory pathophysiology. Chest 83:666–670, 1983.

Murray IP, Modell JH: Early detection of endotracheal tube accidents by monitoring carbon dioxide concentration in respiratory gas. Anesthesiology 59:344–346, 1983.

Jerry IP, Modell JH, Gallagher TJ, et al.: Titration of PEEP by the arterial minus end-tidal carbon dioxide gradient. Chest 85:100–104, 1984.

Jordan L, Huffman LM: Monitoring in anesthesia; Clinical application of monitoring oxygenation and ventilation. J Am Assoc Nurse Anesthesiol 53:513–525, 1985.

Birmingham PK, Cheney FW, Ward RJ: Esophageal intubation; A review of detection techniques. Anesth Analg 1986.

Cheng EY, Renschler MF, Mihm FG, et al.: Non-invasive respiratory monitoring of patients during weaning from mechanical respiratory support. Anesth Analg 65:S29, 1986.

Shafieha MJ, Sit J, Kartha R, et al.: End-tidal CO_2 analyzers in proper positioning of the doublelumen tubes. Anesthesiology 64:844–845, 1986.

Selby DG, Ilsley AH, Runciman WB: An evaluation of five carbon dioxide analyzers for use in the operating theatre and intensive care unit. Anesthesiol Intens Care 15:212–216, 1987.

Sharer K, Sladen R: Ventilator management by pulse oximetry and capnometry after cardiac surgery. Anesthesiology 69:A27, 1988.

Stock MC: Noninvasive carbon dioxide monitoring. Critical Care Clinics 4:511–526, 1988.

Griffis CA: End-tidal CO_2 monitoring during anesthesia. J Am Assoc Nurse Anesthesiol 54:312–318, 1986.

Garnett AR, Ornato JP, Gonzalez ER, et al.: End-tidal carbon dioxide monitoring during cardiopulmonary resuscitation. JAMA 257:512–515, 1987.

Healey CJ, Fedullo AJ, Swinburne AJ, et al.: Comparison of noninvasive measurements of carbon dioxide tension during withdrawal from mechanical ventilation. Crit Care Med 15:764–768, 1987.

Harris K: Noninvasive monitoring of gas exchange. Respir Care 32:544–553, 1987.

Phan CQ, Tremper KK, Lee SE, et al.: Noninvasive monitoring of carbon dioxide; A comparison of the partial pressure of transcutaneous end-tidal carbon dioxide with the partial pressure of arterial carbon dioxide. J Clin Monit 3:149–154, 1987.

Lepilin MG, Vasilyev AV, Bildinow OA, et al.: End-tidal carbon dioxide as a noninvasive monitor of circulatory status during cardiopulmonary resuscitation; A preliminary clinical study. Crit Care Med 15:958–959, 1987.

Niehoff J, DelGuerico C, LaMorte W, et al.: Efficacy of pulse oximetry and capnometry in postoperative ventilatory weaning. Crit Care Med 16:701–705, 1988.

Mogue LR, Rantala B: Capnometers. J Clin Monit 4:115–121, 1988.

Marini JJ: Monitoring during mechanical ventilation. Clin Chest Med 9:73–100, 1988.

Dunphy JA: Accuracy of expired carbon dioxide partial pressure sampled from a nasal cannula. Anesthesiology 68:960–961, 1988.

Lillie PE, Robertg JG: Carbon dioxide monitoring Anesth Intens Care 16:41–44, 1988.

Gudipati CV, Weil MH, Bisera J, et al.: Expired carbon dioxide, a noninvasive monitor cardiopulmonary resuscitation. Circulation 77:234–239, 1988.

Leasa DJ, Sibbald WJ: Respiratory monitoring in a critical care unit. Curr Pulmonol 9:209–265, 1988.

Carlon GC, Ray C, Miodownik S, et al.: Capnography in mechanically ventilated patients. Crit Care Med 16:550–556, 1988.

Guggenberger H, Lenz G, Federle R: Early detection of inadvertent oesophageal intubation, Pulse oximetry vs. capnography. Acta Anaesthesiol Scand 33:112–115, 1989.

Hoffman RA, Krieger BP, Kramer MR, et al.: End-tidal carbon dioxide in critically ill patients during changes in mechanical ventilation. Am Rev Respir Dir 140:1265–1268, 1989.

Bowe EA, Boysen PG, Broome JA, et al.: Accurate determination of end-tidal carbon dioxide during administration of oxygen by nasal cannulae. J Clin Monit 5:105–110, 1989.

Sanders AB, Kern KB, Otto CW, et al.: End-tidal carbon dioxide monitoring during cardiopulmonary resuscitation; A prognostic indicator for survival. JAMA 262:1347–1351, 1989.

Morley TF: Capnography in the intensive care unit. J Intens Care Med 5:209–223, 1990.

Russell GB, Graybeal JM: Stability of arterial to end-tidal carbon dioxide gradients during postoperative cardiorespiratory support. Can J Anesthesiol 37:560–566, 1990.

11.0 GLOSSARY

Acinus — A group of alveoli in the lower airway of the lung that forms a functional respiratory unit supplying gas and blood for respiration.

Airway resistance — Resistance specific to the movement of air through the conducting airways beginning at the mouth and/or nose and continuing through the large bronchi, the bronchioles, and ending in the alveoli. For patients on mechanical ventilators, airway resistance includes the resistance of the ventilator circuitry and the endotracheal tube.

Alveolar macrophages — A specific type of blood cells found in the alveoli that aids in sequestering and destroying bacteria.

Alveoli — The tiny air sacs at the end of the airways in the lung; composed of very thin flat cells that form the network for gas exchange between fresh air and venous blood.

Anemometer — An instrument for measuring the force and speed of air through a medium such as lung tissue.

Angle of Louis — The slight angle that exists between the manubrium and the body of the sternum.

Apnea — A transient stoppage of breathing.

Avogadro's law — The principle that equal volumes of different gases under identical conditions of pressure and temperature contain the same number of molecules.

Base impedance —The base value of impedance used for both children and adult electrocardiogram electrodes; usually around 500 Ohms.

Bicarbonate — The chemical radical group denoted by HCO3 or a compound containing this group; bicarbonate acts as a buffer to absorb hydrogen or other kinds of ions.

Blood resevoir — A function of the lung in that it serves as a receiving chamber for venous blood returning to the right ventricle of the heart.

Boyles's law —The principal that at a fixed temperature, the pressure of a confined ideal gas varies inversely with its volume.

Bronchus — Bronchi, plural; any of the larger air passages of the lungs having an outer fibrous coat with irregularly placed plates of hyaline cartilage, an interlacing of smooth muscle, and a mucous membrane of columnar epithelial cells.

Capacitance — The proportionality constant relating the electric charge of a device that stores electric energy to the voltage across the two conductive elements of the device.

Capnography — The graphic representation and interpretation of the waveform of the changing concentration of carbon dioxide during the entire respiratory cycle.

Capnometers — Instruments developed to record and interpret the waveform of the changing concentration of carbon dioxide during the entire respiratory cycle.

Carbon dioxide transport — The elimination of carbon dioxide, the byproduct of cellular metabolism, from the capillary venous blood via the lungs.

Carbonic anhydrase — An enzymatic protein in the blood that acts as a catalyst to enhance certain chemical reactions in the blood.

Cardiac arrhythmia — An alteration of either time or force of the rhythm of the heartbeat.

Cardiac diastole — The dilation or period of dilation of a chamber of the heart.

Carboxyhemoglobin — The hemoglobin molecule that combines with carbon dioxide when transporting it through the lungs for removal from the ventilatory system.

Cardiac output — The volume of blood pumped by the heart per unit time, usually expressed in liters per minute (l/min); also the product of the heart rate and the stroke volume.

Cardiac systole — The contraction or period of contraction of the heart or one of its chambers.

Cerebrospinal fluid (CSF) — The serumlike fluid that bathes the lateral ventricles of the brain and the cavity of the spinal cord.

c' flow — The measurement of the oxygenation of the end-pulmonary capillary blood.

Charles' law — The physical law that the volume of a fixed mass of gas held at a constant pressure varies directly with the absolute temperature (also related to Gay-Lussac's law).

Chemical receptors — (Also, chemoreceptors). A protein molecule usually found at a nerve ending or in a sense organ such as for smell or taste that is sensitive to chemical stimulation.

Chloride shift — The reaction across the cellular membrane that promotes the movement of bicarbonate ions out of the cell in exchange for chloride ions from the plasma into the cell; maintains electrical and chemical equilibrium in the system.

Compliance — A measure of how easily the lung distends when a gas passes through; the reciprocal of elasticity.

Cough mechanism — A function of the larynx; clears particles from the larynx, trachea, and large airways; operates in several phases including irritation,deep inspiration, airway closure, compression, airway opening, and expulsion.

Dalton's law of partial pressures — This law states that each gas in a mixture contributes its share of the total pressure in proportion to its percentage or concentration in the mixture.

Deadspace gas — The amoung of gas left in the conducting airways at the end of the breath or gas that reaches capillaries with no blood supply.

Diaphragm — A primary muscle in the abdomen that elongates the thoracic cavity during inspiration and is innervated by the right and left phrenic nerves from the spinal cord.

Diffusion — The movement of gases across a membrane and into and out of cells due to their tendency to move from areas of higher kinetic energy to areas of lower kinetic energy or concentration.

Diffusion coefficient — A special factor used in determining the rate of diffusion across a membrane; see Fick's principle or law.

Diffusion impairment — Occurs when the alveolar capillary membrane becomes thickened (for example, in pulmonary edema) and results from ventilation perfusion inequality.

Dynamic ventilation — A complex set of functions, including muscle movement resulting in changes in size and shape of the thorax and lung, cyclic pressure changes in the thorax and lung leading to gas movement and volume change, and gas distribution within the lung as related to compliance and resistance.

Dyshemoglobins — Faulty, incorrect, malformed hemoglobin.

Elasticity — A measure of the force with which the lung fibers attempt to recoil after deflation; the reciprocal of compliance.

Electrocardiogram (ECG or EKG) — The signal traced by an electrocardiograph; used to diagnose heart disease that modifies the electrical activity of the heart.

Electrochemical sensors — Devices to routinely measure inspiratory oxygen in patient vetilator circuits; include polarographic types and galvanic or fuel cell types.

Epiglottis — The section of tissue, located at the superior musculature of the larynx, that covers and protects the airway from the aspiration of food particles or foreign bodies during swallowing.

Expiratory cycle (Te) — The expiratory component of the ventilatory cycle controlled by the expiratory neurons in the medulla of the brainstem.

Expiratory reserve volume (ERV) — The amount of volume exhaled forcefully from the resting position when the lung and thorax exert equal forces.

External respiration — The exchange of gas that occurs at the alveolar capillary level of the lung and exchanges oxygen supplied from the atmosphere by ventilation and the venous blood supplied by the lung capillaries.

Fick Principle — (Also as Fick's law). The rate of diffusion of a gas across a membrane is proportional to the surface area of the membrane, a diffusion coefficient, the partial pressure differences or concentration difference between the two sides of the membrane.

Forced expiratory volume (FEV) — The amount of air forced out of the lung.

Functional residual capacity (FRC) — The amount of gas in the lung when the lung elastic forces and the thoracic forces are equal but pulling in opposite directions.

Functional saturation (%SaO$_2$) — The sum of the oxygen saturation of the four hemoglobin species in the blood.

Galvanic cell sensor — Used to measure inspiratory oxygen in the patient ventilation circuit with an electrochemical cell; has a gold or platinum cathode and a lead or copper anode with potassium hydroxide as the usual electrolyte.

Gas exchange — The interchange of essential oxygen and the waste product of metabolism, carbon dioxide, as well as other minor gases by the respiratory system in the lung.

Gay-Lussac's law — The physical law that the volume of a fixed mass of gas held at a constant pressure varies directly with the absolute temperature (see Charles's law).

General Gas law — Also Ideal Gas law; states that the pressure and the volume of a gas relates to the number of gas molecules present and the absolute temperature multiplied by a gas constant.

Glottis — The opening through which air enters the airway.

Graham's law — This principle states that the relative rates of diffusion of gases under the same conditions are inversely proportional to the square roots of the molecular weight(s) of the gas(es); an application of the kinetic theory of gases.

Hemoglobin — The iron-containing protein in red blood cells that carries oxygen.

Henry's law — This principle states that the quantity of gas that dissolves in a liquid is proportional to the partial pressure and solubilities of each gas.

Hering-Breuer reflex — The reflex from the prolongation of the respiratory cycle produced by maintaining lung inflation.

Humidity determination — Measurement of water vapor in the humidified gas delivered by modern ventilators by specific humidity sensors.

Hypercarbia — Excess carbon dioxide in the blood; also hypercapnia.

Hypopnea — Abnormally slow and shallow breathing.

Hypoventilation — The underventilation of the lung; causes fresh oxygen not to be replenished in the lung so that arterial oxygen tensions start to approach those of venous blood and reduced the partial pressure gradient between the gas and the blood.

Hypoxemia — Deficiency of oxygen in the blood; also hypoxia.

Immunoglobulins — A class of protein molecules that act as antibodies to immobilize certain bacteria and viruses.

Impedance — A measure of the total opposition to current in a circuit or air through an airway.

Inertia — Forces required to accelerate the gas and tissues making up the respiratory system. During normal breathing, inertia remains negligible.

Infrared spectrophotometry — A measurement system based on the principle that different gases absorb infrared light at different wavelengths.

Inspiration — The intake of air into the lungs; occurs when alveolar pressure falls below the atmospheric pressure; a form of negative breathing.

Inspiratory cycle — The inspiratory component of the ventilatory cycle under the control of the inspiratory neurons at the end of nerves from the medulla of the brainstem.

Inspiratory reserve volume (IRV) — The maximum amount of air that can be inhaled following a normal quiet inspiration.

Intermittent positive pressure breathing (IPPB) — Also called mechanical ventilation; the situation in which the alveolar pressure causes the capillary to collapse.

Internal respiration — The gas exchange occurring between the systemic capillary cells and the actual tissue cells; at this level, the oxygen need and the carbon dioxide removal depends on the metabolic activity of the cells.

Intrapleural pressure — The pressure surrounding the lung.

Irritant receptors — Nerve endings located primarily in the upper airways that respond to changes in lung volume during inspiration and expiration.

Juxtacapillary receptors (J receptors) — Nerve endings located close to the pulmonary capillary; they respond to capillary congestion as seen in pulmonary edema and to certain types of drugs.

Kinetic theory of gases — The theory of gas behavior that states a gas that occupies a space is not continuous, gas molecules are in constant motion and have kinetic energy, and gas molecules continually collide with one another.

Laryngopharynx — The section of the upper airway from the base of the tongue to the opening of the esophagus; contains the glottis, the opening through which air enters the airway and the epiglottis which covers and protects the airway during swallowing.

Larynx — The cartilaginous, connective passage way between the upper and lower airways that functions to house the vocal cords.

Laser-doppler anemometer — An instrument used to measure the force and speed of air through the lung tissue using real-time integration of flow and volume measurements.

Lung clearance — The ability of the lung to mechanically and chemically clear itself of inhaled foreign particles.

Lung compliance — The measure of how easily the lung distends.

Lung parenchyma — The lung tissue surrounding, but not connected to, the bronchi.

Macrophages — A type of blood cells that sequester and rid the blood and tissues of foreign particles or organisms.

Mass spectrometry — The measurement system that uses the relationship between the molecular charge and the mass of substances to determine their concentration in a solution.

Mean arterial pressure (MAP) — The mean blood pressure in the arteries.

Mechanical receptors — Also mechanoreceptors; nerve endings that respond to mechanical factors such as lung volume and muscle tension on the chest wall and diaphragm; they send information back to the respiratory control center to regulate tidal volume and breathing frequency and pulmonary reflexes.

Mechanical ventilation — Aiding or supporting a patient's ventilation using a device to inspire air into the lungs and to extract air from the lungs; used during anesthetic surgery and in intensive care units.

Minute alveolar ventilation (V̇E) — The amount of gas moved in and out of the lung during one minute; also called minute deadspace ventilation.

Mitochondria — The organelle within each cell that contains enzymes to convert food into usable energy.

Mixed venous oxygen saturation (of hemoglobin) — Abbreviated as $S\bar{v}O_2$, a measurement of the oxygen saturation of hemoglobin at the point of oxygen for carbon dioxide exchange; reflects the balance between oxygen delivery and oxygen consumption in the body as a whole.

Motion artifact — The mechanical modulation of the pathlength of the transmitted light due to motion as measured by a pulse oximeter sensor.

Mucociliary blanket — The cells and structures lining the tracheal bronchi that participate in the filtration and clearance of inhaled particles from the lung.

Nares — The external orifices (openings) of the nose.

Ohm's law — A summary of the relations between voltage, current, and resistance whereby voltage equals the product of current and resistance.

Oxyhemoglobin — The combination of oxygen with hemoglobin in an easily reversible reaction.

Partial pressure of oxygen (PO_2) — The pressure that oxygen would exert if it were alone in a container.

Partial pressure of arterial oxygen (PaO_2) — The partial pressure of oxygen in arterial blood.

Partial pressure of venous oxygen (PvO_2) — The partial pressure of oxygen in venous blood, usually determined in venous blood from the pulmonary artery.

Pauling's principle — A phenomenon in which the presence of a magnetic field, oxygen molecules become like small magnets and intensify the strength of the magnetic field.

Perfusion — The flow of blood through the lung, specifically through the pulmonary capillaries; facilitates the diffusion process and serves as the essential carrier mechanism for transport of gases to and from the tissue cells.

Periodic breathing — In infants, the three or more central apneas of at least 3 and or more than 15 seconds long with each separated by no more than 20 seconds of stable regular breathing.

Pharynx — The space behind the oral and nasal cavities; divided into the nasopharynx, the oropharynx, and the larynogopharynx.

Phrenic nerve — The nerve running from the spinal column to the diaphragm that influences the total ventilatory cycle, including the inspiratory and the expiratory components.

Photoplethysmography — A system of measurement that differentiates arterial from venous blood using light reflectance or light transmission through vascular tissue to measure arterial pressure waveforms generated by the cardiac cycle.

Pitot tube — An older device used to measure pressure differences across a known resistance during gas movement; consists of a tube with a short right-angled bend that orients vertically in the stream of gas so that the end is directed up stream.

Plasma proteins — Proteins that reside in the blood (serum) and that bind to various kinds of gases, thus acting as carrier molecules in the human circulatory system.

Pleura — The serous membrane interspersed throughout the lungs and lining of the thoracic cavity. It completely encloses a potential space known as the pleural cavity.

Pneumocytes, alveolar — Very flat cells approximately one tenth of a micron in thickness that make up the alveolus (alveoli, plural), the primary functional gas exchange unit.

Pneumothorax — The accumulation of air in the pleural cavity because of a hole in the lung or chest wall.

Poiseuille's law — The principle that describes the airflow resistance properties of the lung; airflow resistance primarily depends on the physical dimensions of the passages, with the radius being the most important. The pressure required to achieve a constant air flow changes every time the airway geometry changes; thus, resistance equals the pressure difference between peak pressure and plateau pressure divided by airflow.

Polargraphic sensor — Measures inspiratory oxygen in the patient ventilation circuit using an electrochemical cell; uses the ability of oxygen to chemically react with water in the presence of electrons to produce hydroxyl ions.

Premature ventricular contractions (PVCs) — Signals seen on electrocardiograms that indicate the premature contractions of the ventricle of the heart.

Pulmonary blood flow — The blood flow achieved through the branching network of pulmonary arteries that distribute venous blood to the alveolar capillaries of gas exchange and to the secondary perfusion system of the smaller bronchial arteries.

Pulmonary circulation — The blood system in the lung, which comprises two main pulmonary arteries, branching into the bronchi, and finally forming the sheet-like capillary network called the alveolar capillary.

Pulmonary stretch receptors — Nerve endings that receive input by the stretch of the lung smooth muscles; they are sensitive to stretch as lung volume or pressure changes.

Pulse oximetry — A noninvasive method to measure the color of the hemoglobin molecule, and therefore oxygen saturation of the arterial blood, through the skin.

Pulse oximeter — Instruments that measure patient ventilation using a pulse waveform continuous monitoring system.

Raman spectrometry — A measurement system based on the Raman effect in which scattering occurs when photons from a laser beam collide with gas molecules.

Residual volume (RV) — The amount of air remaining in the lung after a complete exhalation.

Resistance — Opposition or counter-acting force; an impediment to air flow through the tissue.

Respiratory signal ΔZ — The vector composed of capicitative and resistive impedance.

Shunt — The situation when blood bypasses the lung; shunted blood does not undergo an exchange with alveolar gas and has a lowered arterial oxygen tension below that of the alveoli.

Spectrophotometry — A system of measurement of the hemoglobin saturation based on the color and optical density of the hemoglobin molecule.

Spirometer — A device to measure lung volumes and ventilation; includes a breathing tube, a collection chamber, and a calibrated recording device.

Starling resistor phenomenon — The blood flow in the second zone of perfusion of the lung at the level of the alveoli where the amount of blood flow depends on the difference between the arterial perfusion pressure and the air or alveolar pressure.

Tidal volume (V_T) — The volume of gas moved during normal restful breathing.

Tissue viscous resistance — The frictional resistance caused by movement of the tissues of the lung and the chest wall.

Trachea — The tubular structure of the lower airway that bifurcates into two mainstem bronchi to conduct air to the right and left lobes of the lung.

Transmittance sensors — A photoreceiver that functions to measure the transmission of light through a monitoring site.

Transpulmonary pressure — The inflating pressure to which the lung unit is exposed; the distending pressures resulting from the effect of gravity on the lung.

Ventilation — the movement of air in and out of the chest; includes the movement or changes in both the thoracic cage and the lung.

Ventilation perfusion ratio — The ratio that determines the amounts of oxygen and carbon dioxide exchanged in each unit.

Ventilatory cycle — The complete cycle of inspiration and expiration of gases controlled by the medulla of the brainstem; regulated primarily by negative feedback mechanisms.

Wheatstone bridge — An instrument or circuit consisting of four resistors in series with a galvanometer linking the junction between one pair and the other; used to determine the value of an unknown resistance when the three other resistances are known.

Xiphoid process — The lower end portion of the sternum that is shaped like a sword.

INDEX